CEREBELLUM OF THE RHESUS MONKEY

CEREBELLUM OF THE RHESUS MONKEY

Atlas of Lobules, Laminae, and Folia, in Sections

John C. Madigan, Jr., M.D.
Intern in Surgery
Presbyterian Hospital
New York, N.Y.

and

Malcolm B. Carpenter, M.D.
Professor of Anatomy
College of Physicians and Surgeons
Columbia University
New York, N.Y.

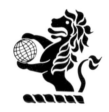

UNIVERSITY PARK PRESS
BALTIMORE · LONDON · TOKYO

Library of Congress Catalog Card Number 76-144388
International Standard Book Number (ISBN) 0-8391-0593-2
Copyright © 1971 by University Park Press
All Rights Reserved
Printed in the United States of America

Contents

Acknowledgments

This project was supported by a research grant (NS–01538–12) from the National Institute of Neurological Diseases and Stroke of the National Institutes of Health, Bethesda, Maryland.

Dr. John C. Madigan, Jr., was supported by training grant 5T01–NS 05242–11 from the National Institute of Neurological Diseases and Stroke.

The authors are pleased to acknowledge the valuable assistance of Mr. Antonio B. Pereira (photography), Mr. Robert J. Demarest (art work), Mrs. Greta Katzauer (histology) and Mrs. Ruth Gutmann (secretary) whose important contributions made this atlas possible.

Introduction

In spite of a wealth of histological detail concerning the structural organization of the cerebellar cortex (Cajal, 1909–1911; Scheibel and Scheibel, 1954; Bell and Dow, 1967; Fox, Hillman, Siegesmund, and Dutta, 1967) and impressive physiological studies (Eccles, Ito, and Szentágothai, 1967) of its neuronal machinery, precise anatomical localization within the various lobules continues to present problems. While certain surface localizations can be made readily from gross specimens, these are limited because many folia do not extend to exposed surfaces. Precise identification of cerebellar lobules and folia can be made only in serial microscopic preparations. However, even in serial sections of the cerebellum, topographical orientation and localization are not easy, except in certain planes. The lobules of the cerebellar vermis can be identified readily in midsagittal sections but are more difficult to identify in serial sections cut transversely or horizontally. Likewise, sagittal sections through the cerebellar hemisphere present problems in identification because prominent landmarks are lacking, or appear different. In the cerebral cortex different areas possess distinctive cytoarchitectonic features which facilitate localization in histological preparations, but the uniform structural organization of the cerebellar cortex provides no unique localizing features. Recognition of this problem in neuropathology led to the preparation of a detailed atlas of the human cerebellum (Angevine, Mancall, and Yakovlev, 1961). While there are important descriptions of the monkey cerebellum (Bolk, 1906; Riley, 1928; Larsell, 1953), none of these is sufficiently detailed to serve as an atlas.

The purpose of this study was to prepare a detailed atlas of the lobules, laminae, folia, and fissures of the cerebellum in sagittal, transverse, and horizontal sections, so that investigators using the rhesus monkey would be able to precisely identify any locus within the cerebellar cortex, or the underlying white matter. No attempt was made to present cytological data concerning either the cortex or the deep cerebellar nuclei. A detailed morphological study of the deep cerebellar nuclei in the monkey recognizes four distinct intrinsic nuclei and provides maps and quantitative data (Courville and Cooper, 1970).

Material and Methods

This atlas is based upon eight monkey cerebella which were embedded in paraffin and sectioned serially at 15μ. Sections were cut sagittally and in planes transverse and horizontal to the axis of the brain stem. Every ninth and tenth section was mounted and stained alternately with cresyl violet and by the Weil technique. Two cerebella and brain stems were cut in sagittal and horizontal planes and four were sectioned transversely. From this material three sets of serial sections, one in each plane, were selected for preparing the atlas. Sections in each plane were studied carefully, using gross specimens as a guide to the identification of fissures and lobules. Representative sections in each of the three basic planes were selected at levels where significant changes were occurring. These sections were photographed and enlarged and used as a basis for drawings. In the drawings the deep staining granular layer is represented in black and the position of the various deep cerebellar nuclei is indicated by dashes. The lobules, laminae, folia, and fissures are identified and labelled on each drawing.

The atlas consists of four parts: (1) a series of gross photographs and matched drawings which identify surface structures and provide orientation for the sections of the cerebellum, (2) sagittal, (3) transverse, and (4) horizontal series of photographs and matched drawings which identify nearly all major cerebellar structures seen at low magnifications. The terminology of Larsell (1953) has been used throughout because it is the most authoritative and the most widely accepted.

Description and Terminology

The **cerebellar vermis** is divisible into ten lobules arranged in an orderly sequence and identified by Roman numerals. This convention adopted by Larsell (1952, 1953) as a revision of Bolk's nomenclature has advantages in that homologies can be made between mammals and avian forms. Vermal lobules of the anterior lobe (I–V) are represented by the lingula, central lobule, and the culmen. In each of these lobules major folia on the surface and in the depths of the primary fissure are indicated by lower case letters. In the posterior vermis, lobules VI–IX represent the declive, folium, tuber, pyramis, and uvula. Lobules VII and VIII are each divided into sublobules designated as VIIA, VIIB, VIIIA, and VIIIB. Again most of the major folia are labelled with lower case letters. Note that sublobule VIIB does not extend to the surface. The nodulus, represented by two folia, is designated as lobule X. In some cases, a lobule contains medullary rays which consist of more than one folium. These divisions are called laminae, according to Larsell (1953), and, like folia, are indicated by lower case letters. Examples of the latter are laminae IV_a and IV_b, and V_a and V_b in the anterior vermis.

In addition, in several sections, a single medullary ray appears which is common to two folia. Such a structure is indicated by hyphenated lower case letters, for example, I_{b-c} and V_{d-e} in the anterior vermis.

The **simple lobule** lies on the superior surface of the cerebellum between the primary and posterior superior fissures. According to Larsell (1953), there is considerable variation in the arrangement of minor fissures in the hemispheric extension of the simple lobule. Snider (1952) indicated two surface folia in the hemispheric part of the simple lobule, Hampson, Harrison, and Woolsey (1952) indicated four such folia, while Larsell (1953) found that three superficial folia of lobule VI (vermis) continued laterally to form four surface folia. The basic problem concerns resolving the relationships of the two posterior folia of the hemispheric part of the simple lobule to vermal lobules VI and VIIA. Larsell found that the first hemispheric folium of the simple lobule was formed by the fusion of vermal folia VI_a and VI_b, while the second hemispheric folium represented a lateral continuation of vermal folium VI_c. The two posterior folia of the simple lobule were regarded as direct lateral continuations of vermal folia VI_b and VI_c. However, in some cerebella the two posterior surface folia of the hemispheric simple lobule were connected directly with the base of the folium $VIIA_a$. In such animals the posterior superior fissure was interrupted by a band connecting sublobule $VIIA_a$ with the simple lobule (see Figures 1 and 2). In the cerebella illustrated in this atlas, and in six additional cerebella, folium VIIA$_a$ always extended laterally to form the two posterior surface folia of the hemispheric part of the simple lobule. The two anterior surface folia were formed by lateral continuations of vermal folia VI$_a$, VI$_b$, and VI$_c$ (see Figures 1, 2, 25, 26, 31, and 32).

The **ansiform lobule** lies between the posterior superior fissure and the anso-paramedian fissure (Jansen, 1950). This lobule has three fissures which divide it into four parts. The deepest fissure, the intercrural, separates crus I from crus II. The two or three most rostral folia of crus I (designated as crus I$_a$) are separated from the posterior folia of crus I (designated as crus I$_p$) by intracrural fissure 1. Crus II also is divided by a furrow, designated as intracrural fissure 2. The three most rostral folia of crus II emerge from the posterior wall of the intercrural fissure, extend laterally and become subfoliated. These folia are designated as crus II$_a$. Folia of crus II$_p$ lie ventral to intracrural fissure 2 and lateral to the ansoparamedian fissure which separates these folia from the paramedian lobule; this landmark is not distinct because the ansoparamedian fissure

is not evident on the surface of the cerebellar hemisphere. The ansoparamedian fissure is distinct from the prepyramidal fissure (Figures 19–24). The prepyramidal fissure in the vermis separates the pyramis (VIII) from lobule (VII), while its lateral extension in the hemisphere separates crus II$_p$ from the pars posterior of the paramedian lobule. Crus I and II are connected medially with sublobule VIIA of the vermis.

The **paramedian lobule** consists of those ventromedial folia which lie adjacent to the cerebellar vermis between the prepyramidal fissure and peduncle of the paraflocculus. According to Larsell (1953), this lobule consists of three parts, designated as anterior, posterior, and copular. From a comparative viewpoint, this division is important because in lower forms, such as the rat and cat, the folia of these parts and their vermal connections are prominent. In the monkey these divisions are less distinct and the posterior part is by far the largest. The posterior part in the monkey consists of four elongated folia that extend ventrolaterally on the surface posterior to the prepyramidal fissure. Medially folia of the posterior part

are continuous with the base of sublobule VIIIA.

The anterior part of the paramedian lobule does not reach the surface of the hemisphere; it lies buried in the depths of the fissure separating crus II$_p$ and the posterior part. The two small subsurface folia comprising the anterior part are said to arise from the same medullary core that gives rise to the ansiform lobule. The fissure separating the anterior part of the paramedian lobule from crus II$_p$ is analogous to the ansoparamedian fissure and extends medially to divide lobule VII into sublobules VIIA and VIIB. Therefore the anterior part of the paramedian lobule, its vermal counterpart sublobule VIIB, and the ansoparamedian fissure: (1) are not visible on the cerebellar surface, (2) lie rostral to the prepyramidal fissure and the posterior part of the paramedian lobule, and (3) are related anatomically to the same medullary core that gives rise to the ansiform lobule. It is apparent that there is very little basis for anatomically separating sublobules VIIA and VIIB in the vermis, and crus II and the anterior part of the paramedian lobule in the hemisphere, except that this distinction may be important in a phylogenetic sense. In sagittal sections the ansoparamedian fissure, the two subsurface folia of sublobule VIIB, and its hemispheric extensions, the anterior part of the paramedian lobule, have been identified.

The copular part of the paramedian lobule can be identified caudal to the posterior part as two or three small, short folia adjacent to the peduncle of the paraflocculus. These are the most ventromedial surface folia of the paramedian lobule, and Larsell (1953) considers them to be derived from a medullary core which is continuous with the more caudal regions of the base of vermal sublobule VIIIB. This part of the paramedian lobule is quite distinct in the cat and rat, but is much smaller in the monkey. Although distinguishing the copular part of the paramedian lobule as a separate entity has phylogenetic significance, its small size in the monkey suggests that it might best be considered as a caudal appendage to the posterior part. Both the posterior and copular parts of the paramedian lobule are related by a single medullary core to rostral and caudal parts of the base of vermal lobule VIII.

The **paraflocculus** lies inferior to the paramedian lobule and crus II and dorsal to the flocculus, and has a peduncle, covered by a thin layer of cortex, which issues from the medullary base of vermal lobules VIII and IX. Laterally a series of increasingly longer folia rests on a fibrous band which is continuous medially with the peduncle of the paraflocculus. According to Larsell (1953), the fissure secunda, which separates vermal lobules VIII and IX, can be traced laterally into the hemispheres as a groove which appears to divide the peduncle of the paraflocculus into two parts. In our study it was not possible to identify the hemispheric extension of the fissure secunda, or to distinguish two parts of the peduncle of the paraflocculus. However, relationships of the parafloccular peduncle to the base of ventral lobules VIII and IX were identified. The peduncle of the paraflocculus forms the stalk of both the dorsal and ventral paraflocculus. The dorsal paraflocculus consists of the ten proximal folia while the four distal folia form the ventral paraflocculus. Folia of the dorsal paraflocculus have been identified in sequence by Arabic numerals.

The ventral paraflocculus consists of four folia, the largest and most lateral forming the lobulus petrosus. No attempt was made to study the ventral parafloc-culus in detail because this structure was frequently broken off or traumatized during removal of the brain, or was separated from the dorsal paraflocculus when the cerebella were sectioned. This structure is illustrated in ventral views (Figures 3 and 4) and lateral views (Figures 9 and 10) of the cerebellum.

The **flocculus** lies ventromedial to the paraflocculus and is separated from it by the posterolateral fissure. This lobule consists of ten or eleven folia which arch lateral to the acoustic nerve and the middle cerebellar peduncle and pass upward onto the inferior surface of the cerebellum anteriorly. The peduncle of the flocculus is continuous with the medullary stalk of the nodulus but is difficult to follow as it passes through the inferior medullary velum. It was not possible to precisely identify the peduncle of the flocculus in Nissl preparations, but this band of fibers could be identified grossly and followed rostromedially into the base of the nodulus. The folia of the flocculus are indicated by sequential Arabic numerals (Figures 3, 4, 7, 8, 9, and 10).

Gross Orientation Series

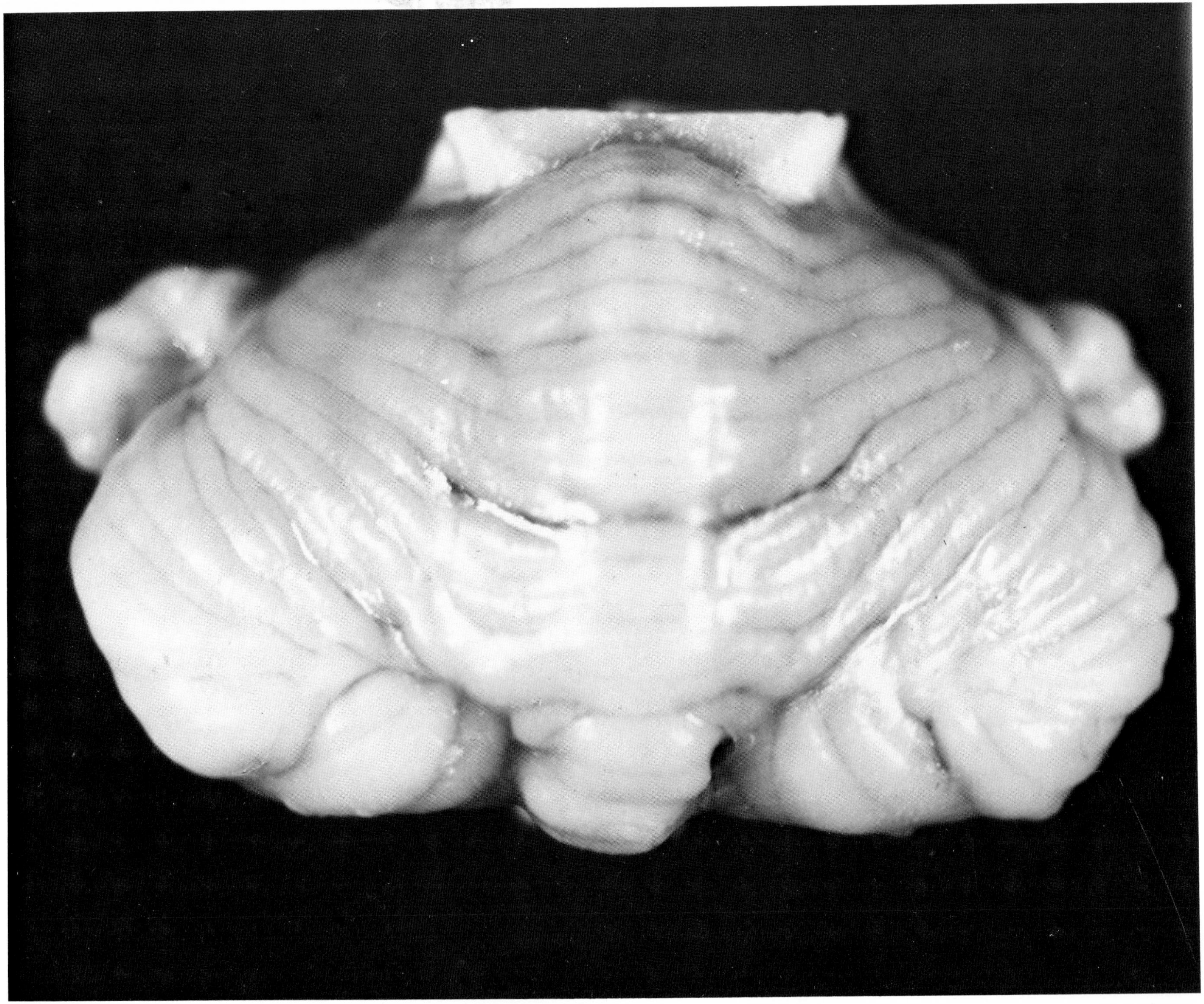

Fig. 1   Photograph of dorsal surface of cerebellum.

14

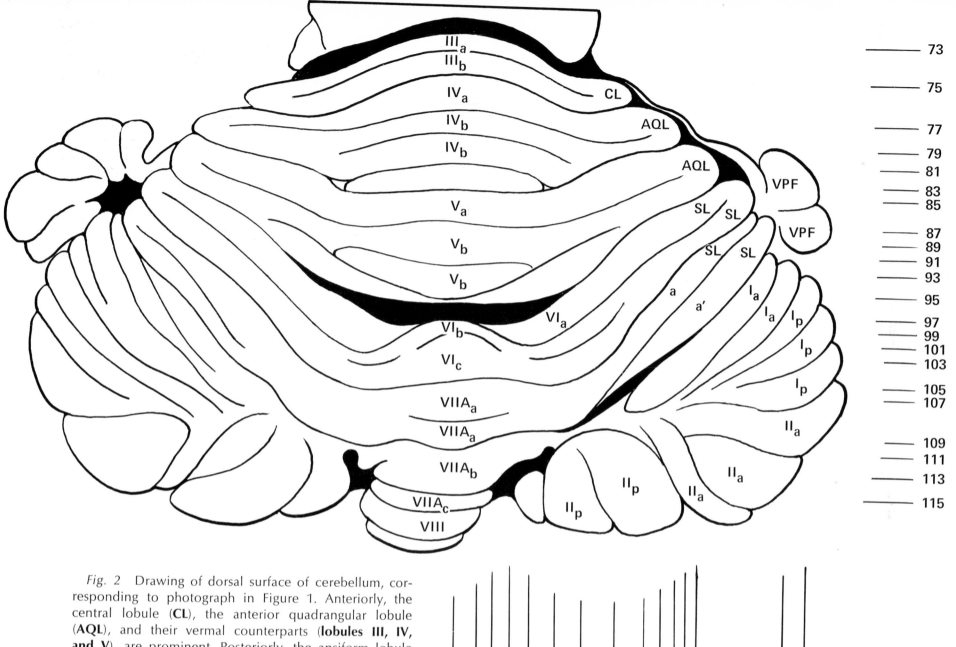

III_a
III_b
IV_a
CL
IV_b
AQL
IV_b
AQL
VPF
V_a
SL SL
VPF
V_b
SL SL
V_b
a a′ I_a
I_a I_p
VI_a
VI_b
I_p
VI_c
I_p
VIIA_a
VIIA_a
II_a
VIIA_b
II_a
II_p II_a
VIIA_c
II_p II_p
VIII

TRANSVERSE SERIES

73
75
77
79
81
83
85
87
89
91
93
95
97
99
101
103
105
107
109
111
113
115

Fig. 2 Drawing of dorsal surface of cerebellum, corresponding to photograph in Figure 1. Anteriorly, the central lobule (**CL**), the anterior quadrangular lobule (**AQL**), and their vermal counterparts (**lobules III, IV, and V**), are prominent. Posteriorly, the ansiform lobule (**crus I_a, I_p, II_a, II_p**) makes up all of the dorsal surface of the hemispheres. The relationship of the four hemispheric folia of the simple lobule (**SL**) to the folia of lobule VI and folium VIIA_a in the vermis, is apparent (cf. Introduction, p. 10; legends for Figures 25–26, and Figures 31–32).

The planes of section of the transverse and sagittal series are indicated and figure numbers of corresponding sections are cited.

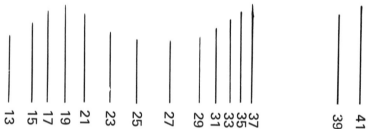

13 15 17 19 21 23 25 27 29 31 33 35 37 39 41

SAGITTAL SERIES

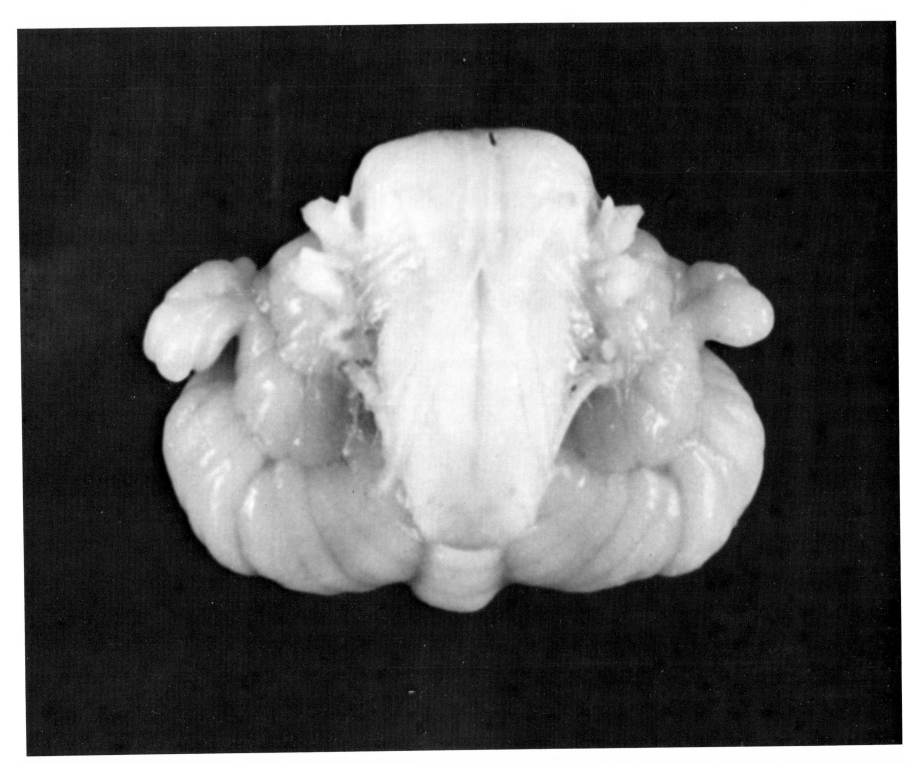

Fig. 3 Photograph of ventral surface of brain stem and cerebellum.

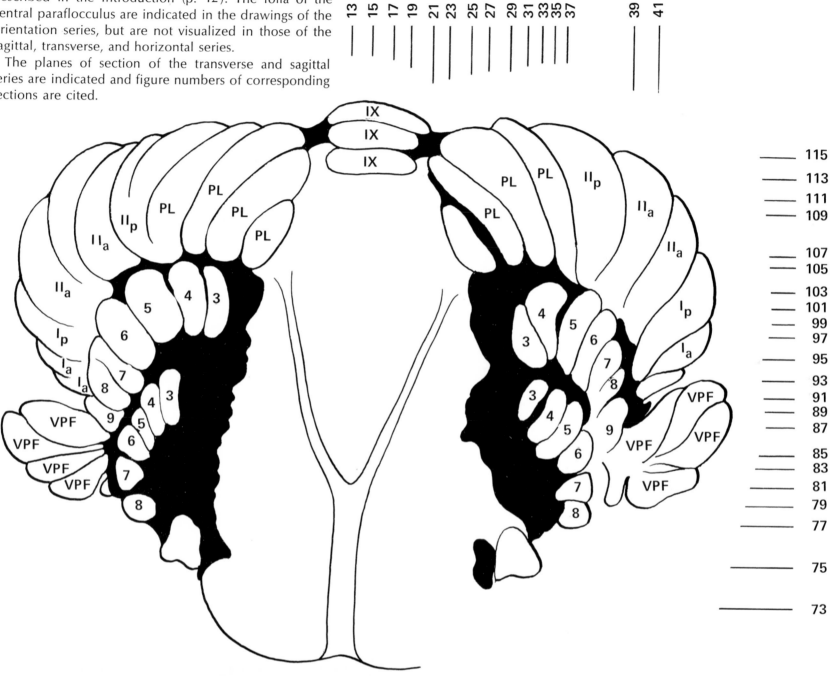

Fig. 4 Drawing of ventral surface of cerebellum, corresponding to photograph in Figure 3. The ventral surfaces of the paramedian lobule (**PL**) and ansiform lobule (**crus I$_a$, I$_p$, II$_a$, II$_p$**) are seen in this view. The folia of the flocculus, and of the dorsal paraflocculus, which lies lateral and posterior to the flocculus, are numbered as described in the Introduction (p. 12). The folia of the ventral paraflocculus are indicated in the drawings of the orientation series, but are not visualized in those of the sagittal, transverse, and horizontal series.

The planes of section of the transverse and sagittal series are indicated and figure numbers of corresponding sections are cited.

SAGITTAL SERIES

13 15 17 19 21 23 25 27 29 31 33 35 37 39 41

TRANSVERSE SERIES

115
113
111
109
107
105
103
101
99
97
95
93
91
89
87
85
83
81
79
77
75
73

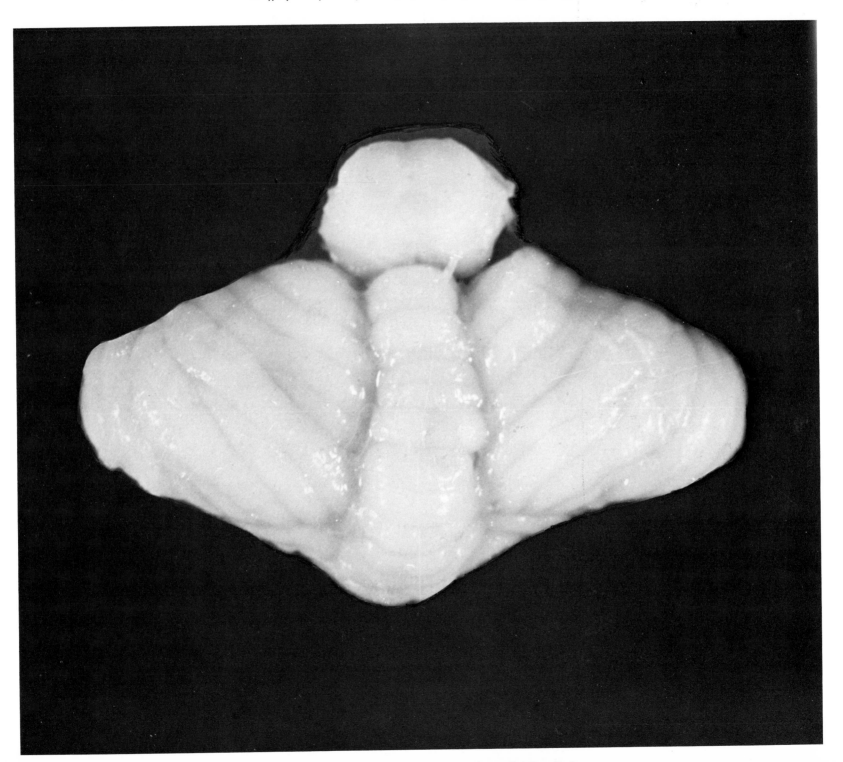

Fig. 5   Photograph of posterior surface of cerebellum.

Fig. 6 Drawing of posterior surface of cerebellum corresponding to photograph in Figure 5. The paramedian lobule (**PL**) and the ansiform lobule (**crus I_p, II_a,** and **II_p**) are prominent in the hemispheres, while lobule VIII and the uvula (**lobule IX**) make up the posterior vermis. The planes of section of the sagittal and horizontal series are indicated and figure numbers of corresponding sections are cited.

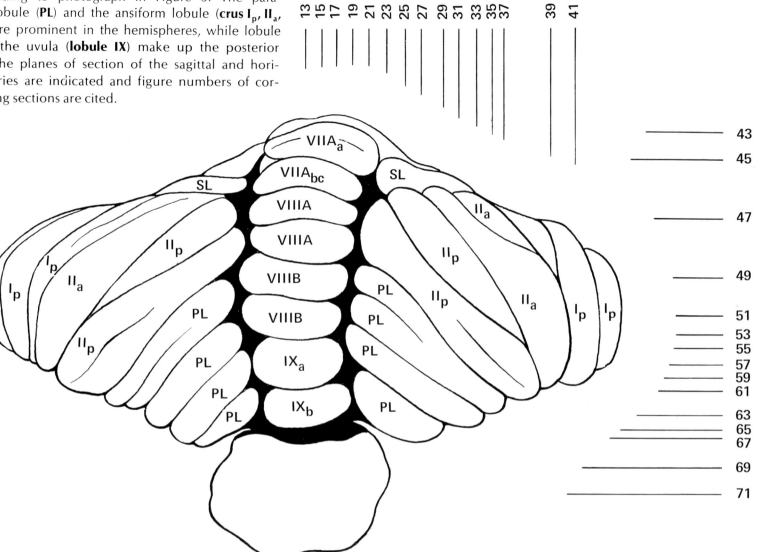

HORIZONTAL SERIES

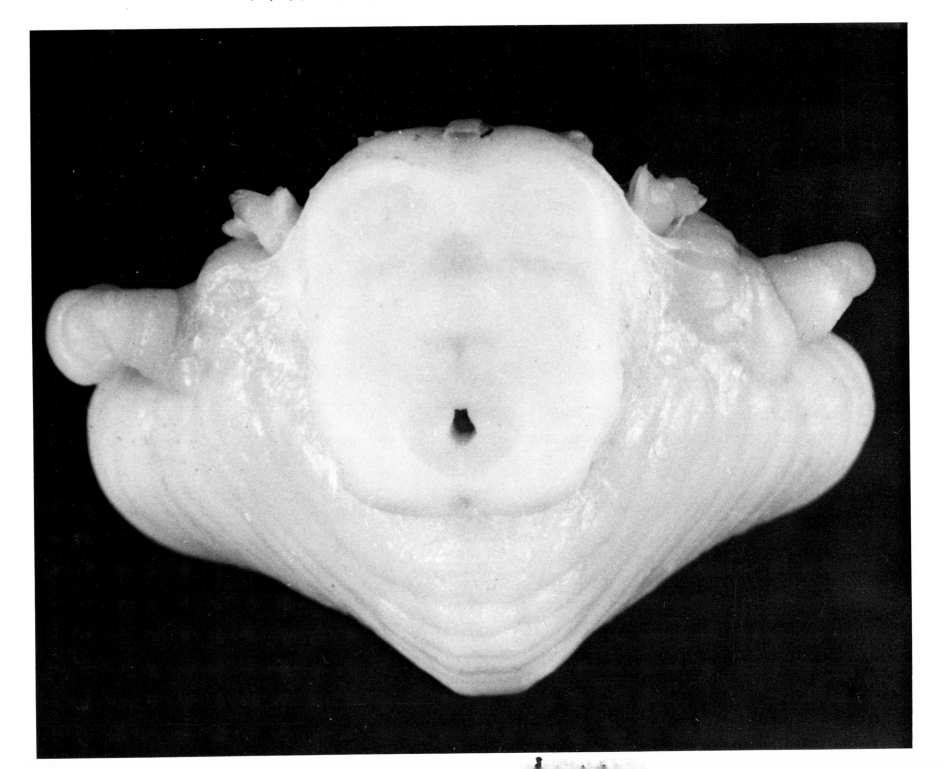

SAGITTAL SERIES

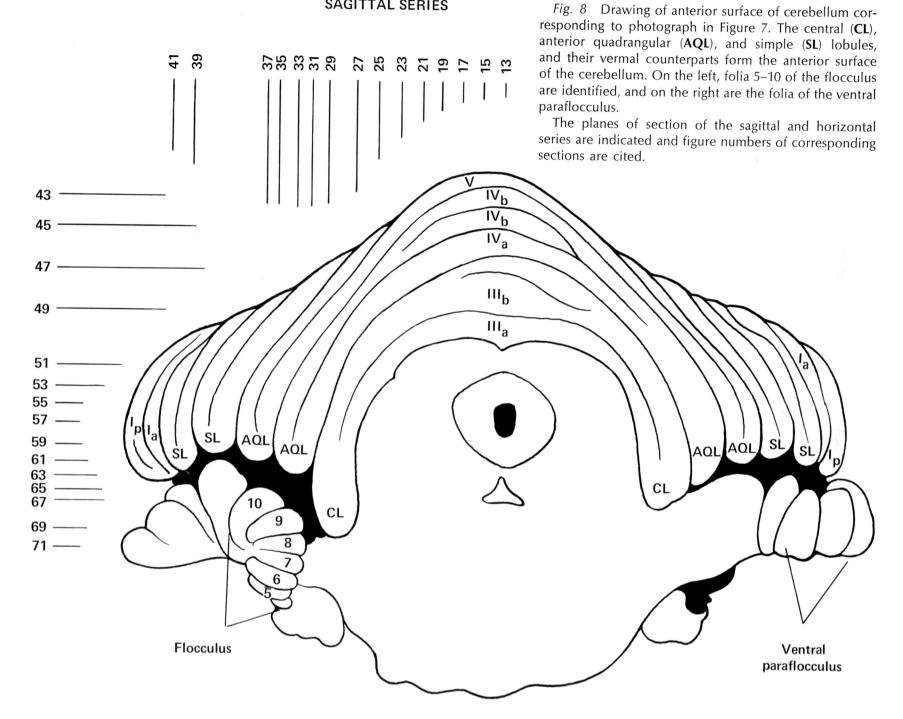

Fig. 8 Drawing of anterior surface of cerebellum corresponding to photograph in Figure 7. The central (**CL**), anterior quadrangular (**AQL**), and simple (**SL**) lobules, and their vermal counterparts form the anterior surface of the cerebellum. On the left, folia 5–10 of the flocculus are identified, and on the right are the folia of the ventral paraflocculus.

The planes of section of the sagittal and horizontal series are indicated and figure numbers of corresponding sections are cited.

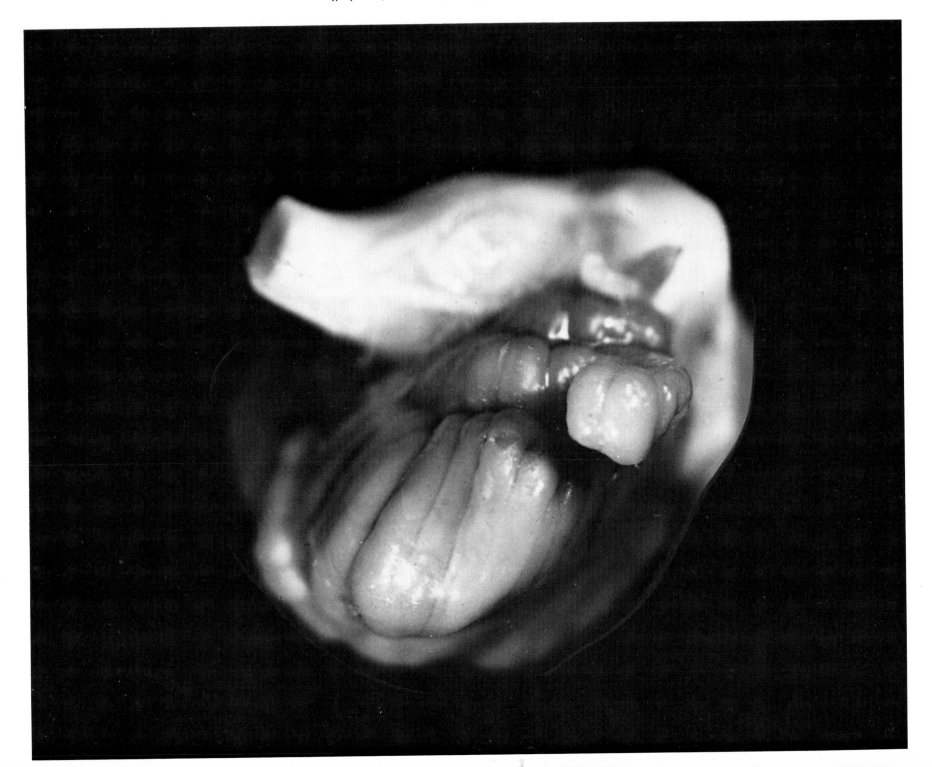

Fig. 9   Photograph of lateral aspect of cerebellum.

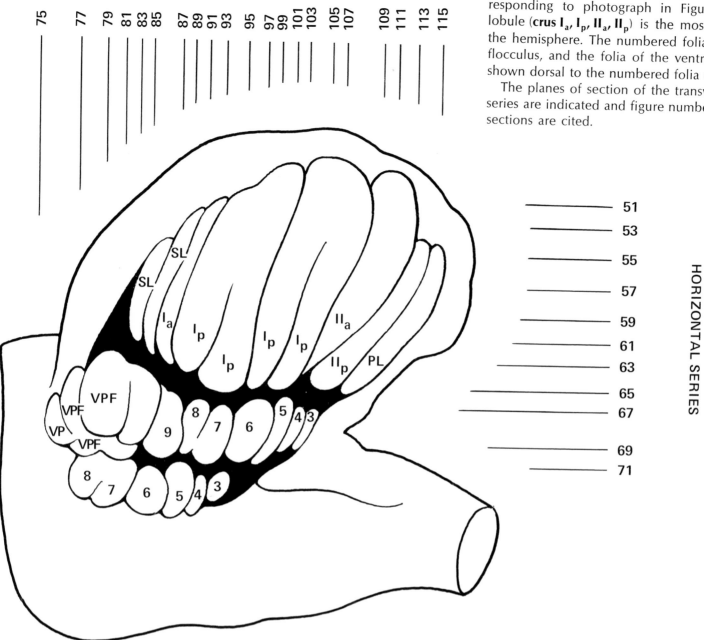

Fig. 10 Drawing of lateral aspect of cerebellum, corresponding to photograph in Figure 9. The ansiform lobule (**crus Ia, Ip, IIa, IIp**) is the most lateral structure in the hemisphere. The numbered folia of the dorsal paraflocculus, and the folia of the ventral paraflocculus, are shown dorsal to the numbered folia of the flocculus.

The planes of section of the transverse and horizontal series are indicated and figure numbers of corresponding sections are cited.

HORIZONTAL SERIES

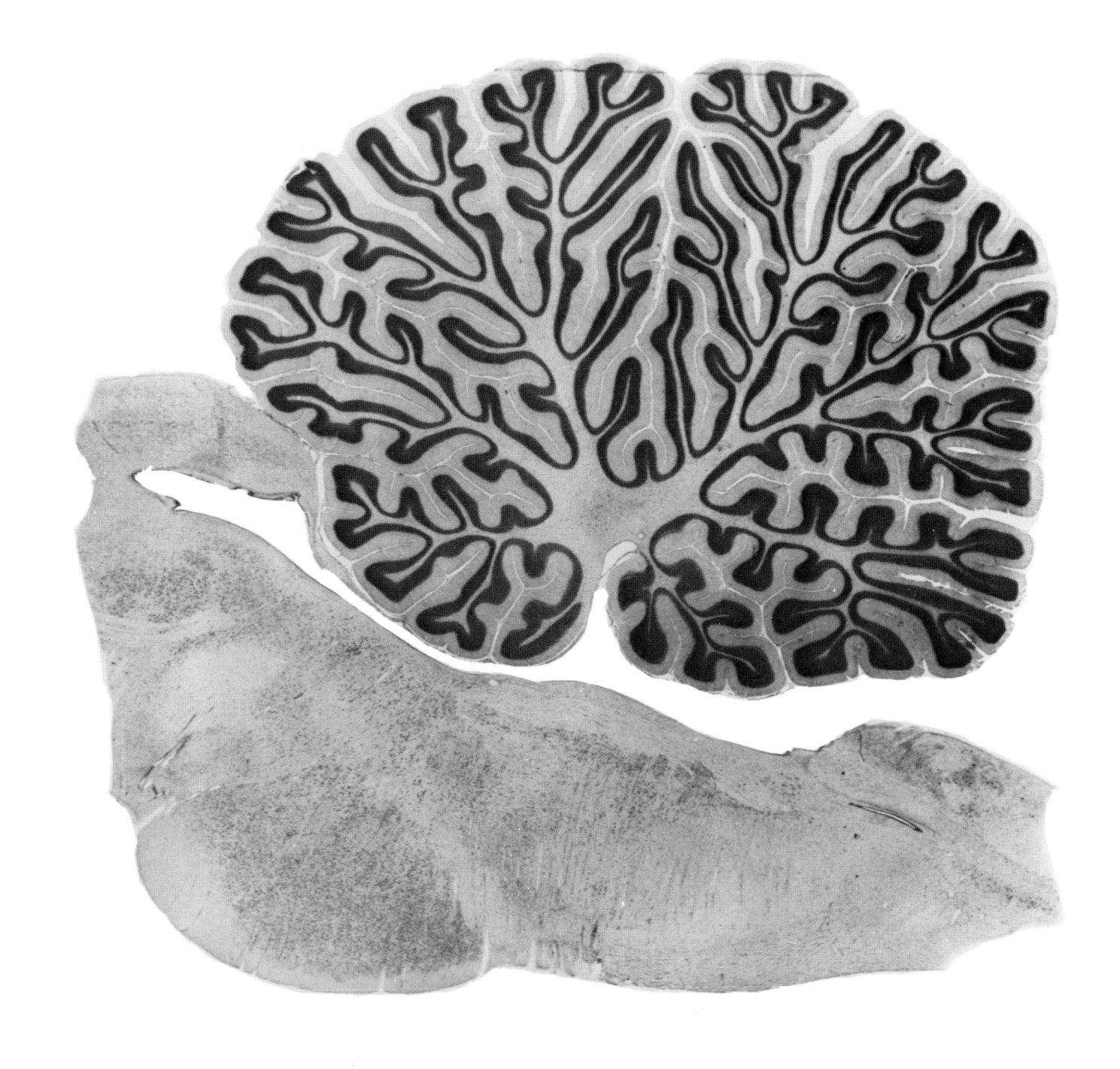

Fig. 11 Photograph of Nissl-stained section through medial cerebellar vermis.

TRANSVERSE SERIES

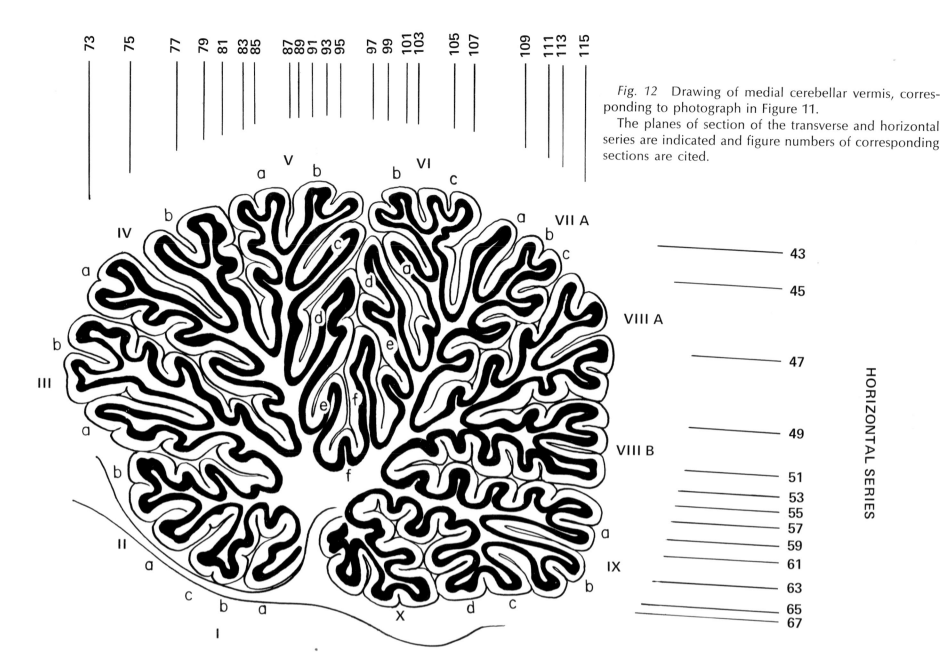

Fig. 12 Drawing of medial cerebellar vermis, corresponding to photograph in Figure 11.
The planes of section of the transverse and horizontal series are indicated and figure numbers of corresponding sections are cited.

HORIZONTAL SERIES

25

Sagittal Section Series

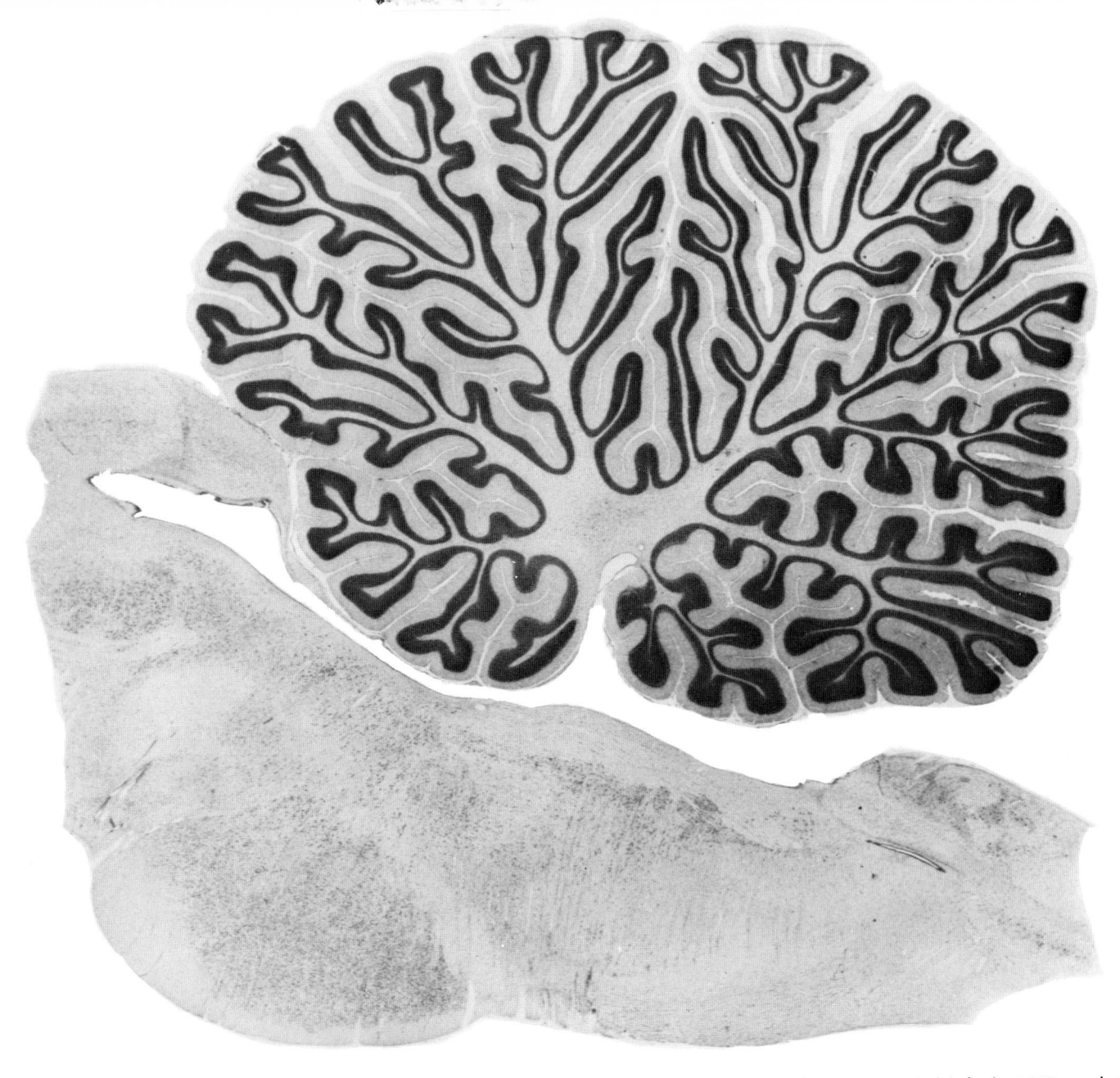

Figs. 13–14 This section lies near the midsagittal plane, as indicated in Orientation Figures 1 through 12. Note the impressive depth of the primary fissure and the large size of the anterior lobe of the cerebellar vermis which contrasts with its relatively small size in the hemispheres. The posterior superior fissure lies between lobules VI and VII, and as described in the Introduction, the ansoparamedian fissure (indicated by **asterisk**) is shown delimiting

sublobule VIIB from VIIA. Sublobule VIIB and the ansoparamedian fissure are not visible on the surface of the cerebellum, but lie in the depths of the prepyramidal fissure. In this plane the fastigial nucleus (**FN**) is prominent. The position and approximate configuration of the deep cerebellar nuclei are indicated in this and succeeding sagittal sections. *Nissl. X 8.*

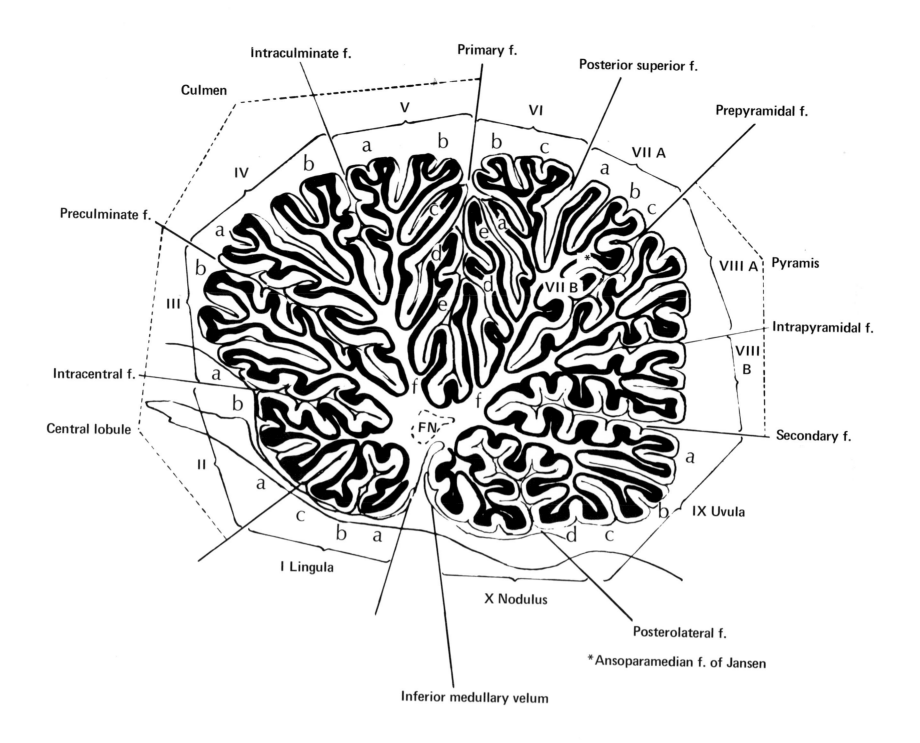

Intraculminate f.

Primary f.

Posterior superior f.

Intracuminate f.

Culmen

Prepyramidal f.

V

VI

VII A

IV

b

b

c

a

Preculminate f.

a

b

a

VIII A

Pyramis

a

c

III

d

b

e

a

VII B

e

d

Intrapyramidal f.

Intracentral f.

a

VIII B

f

Central lobule

b

f

f

FN

Secondary f.

II

a

a

c

IX Uvula

b

a

b

I Lingula

d

c

X Nodulus

Posterolateral f.

*Ansoparamedian f. of Jansen

Inferior medullary velum

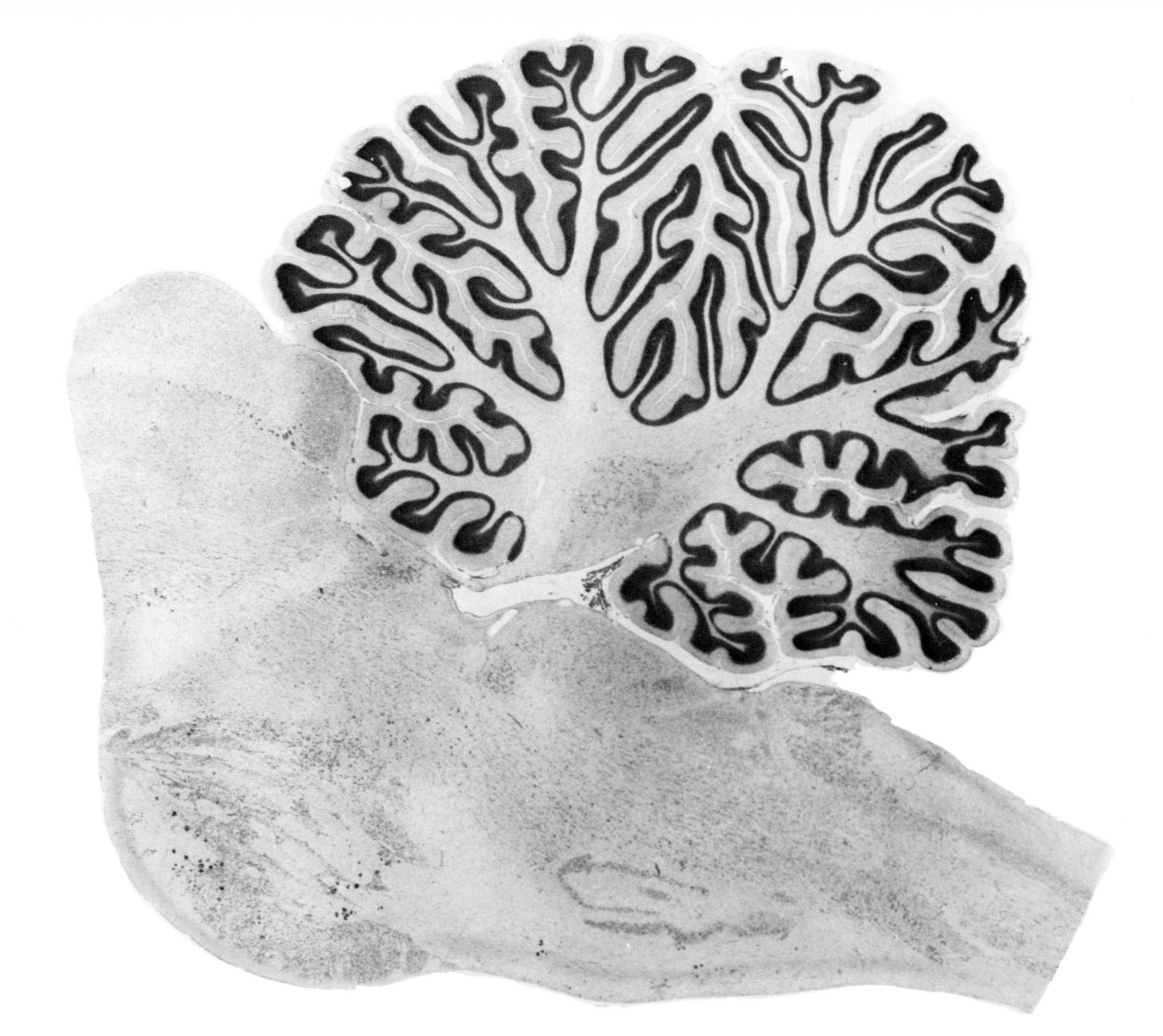

Figs. 15–16 This section is taken through the lateral part of the cerebellar vermis. The lobules and folial pattern are little changed from Figures 13–14, except that folium I_a (**lingula**) is disappearing, the size of the pyramis (**VIIIA** and **VIIIB**) is reduced, and the fastigial nucleus (**FN**) is larger. *Nissl. X 8.*

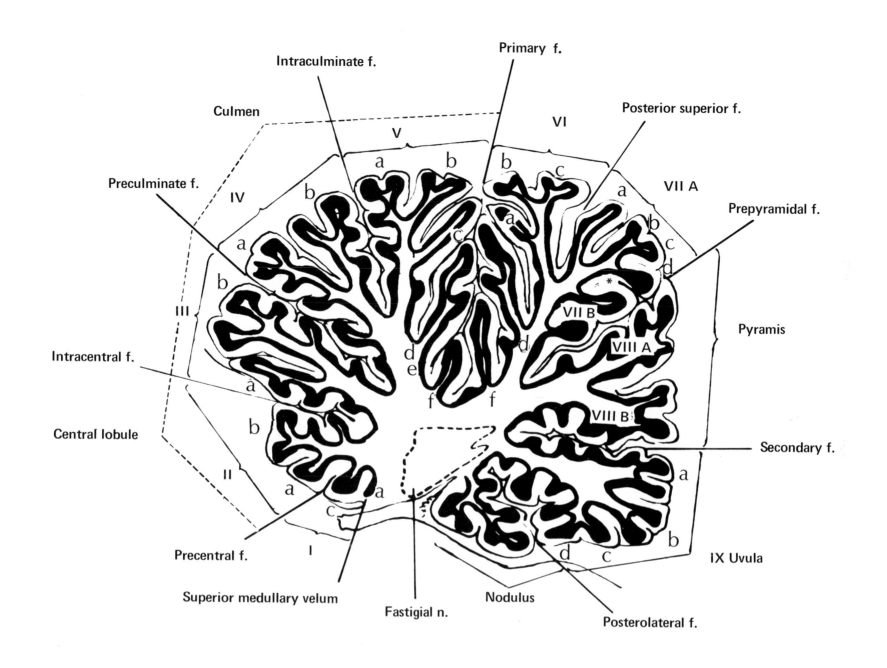

Intraculminate f.

Primary f.

Culmen

Posterior superior f.

V

VI

Preculminate f.

IV

VII A

b

a

b

b

c

Prepyramidal f.

b

a

a

a

III

b

b

c

d

*

VII B

Pyramis

Intracentral f.

a

VIII A

a

d

e

e

f

f

VIII B

Central lobule

b

Secondary f.

II

a

a

a

Precentral f.

I

b

IX Uvula

c

d

c

Superior medullary velum

Nodulus

Fastigial n.

Posterolateral f.

* Ansoparamedian f.

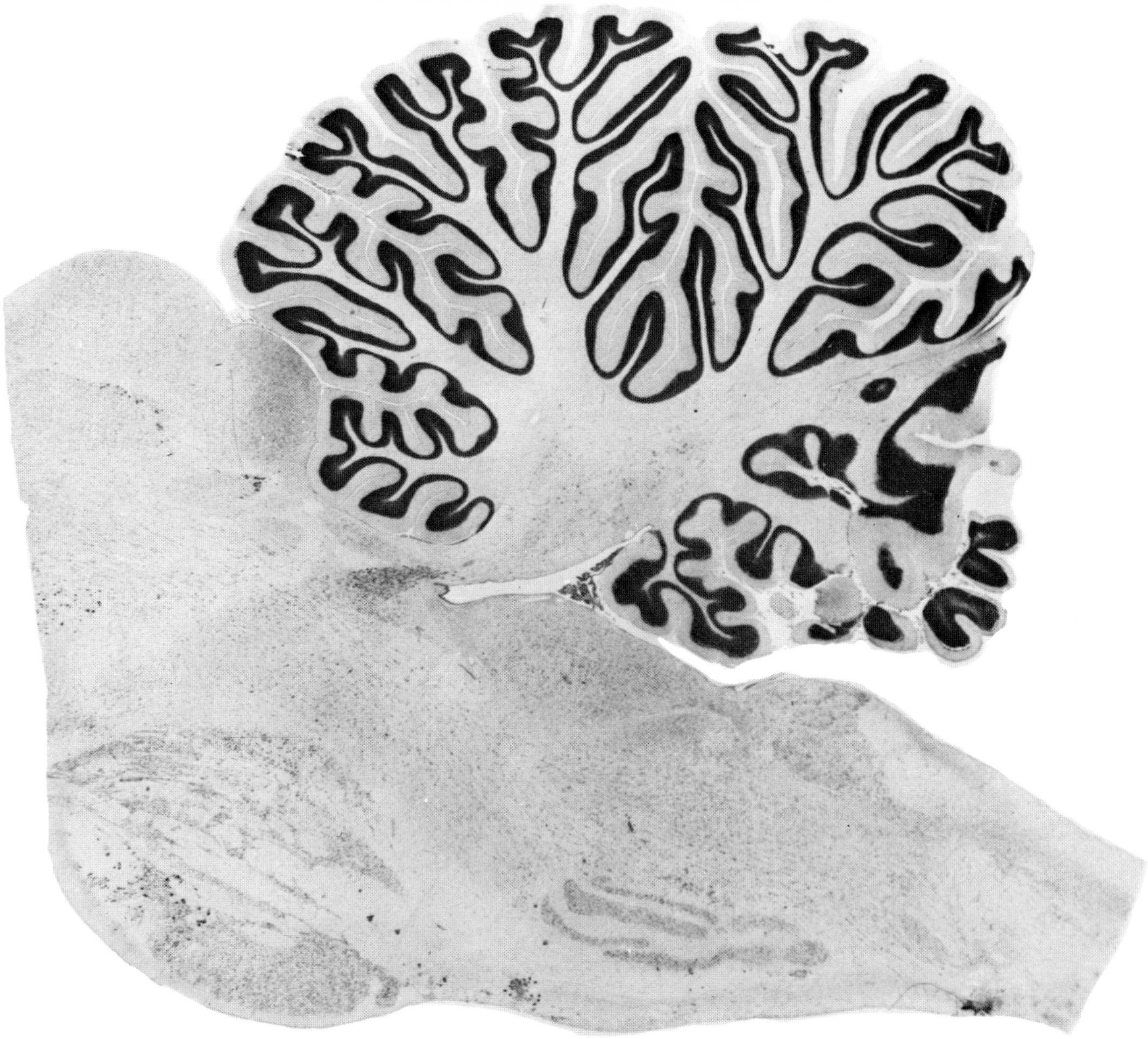

Figs. 17–18 This section is taken through the most lateral part of the vermis and through the depths of the paramedian sulcus separating the posterior vermis from the hemispheres. The nodulus (**lobule X**) extends laterally unchanged. Vermal lobules IX and VIII are greatly reduced, and recognizable mainly by the medullary core at their bases. Sublobules VIIA and VIIB are unchanged, except for the merging of folia VIIA$_b$ and VIIA$_c$. Only folium I$_c$ of the lingula remains. The fastigial nucleus (**FN**) is large, and the medial part of the anterior interposed nucleus has appeared.   *Nissl. X 8.*

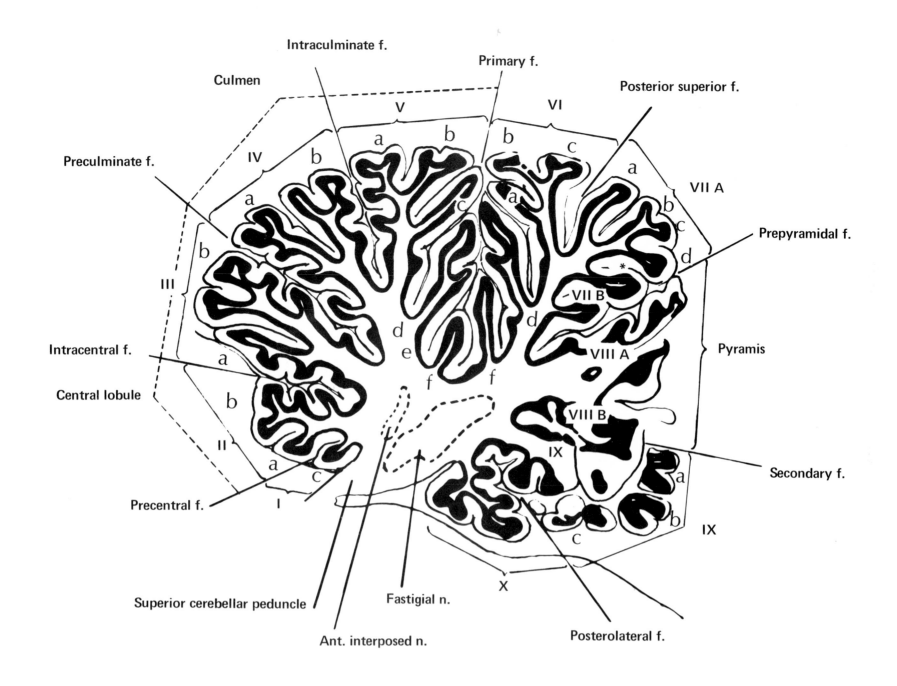

Intraculminate f.

Primary f.

Culmen

Posterior superior f.

Preculminate f.

Prepyramidal f.

Intracentral f.

Pyramis

Central lobule

Secondary f.

Precentral f.

Superior cerebellar peduncle

Fastigial n.

Posterolateral f.

Ant. interposed n.

* Ansoparamedian f.

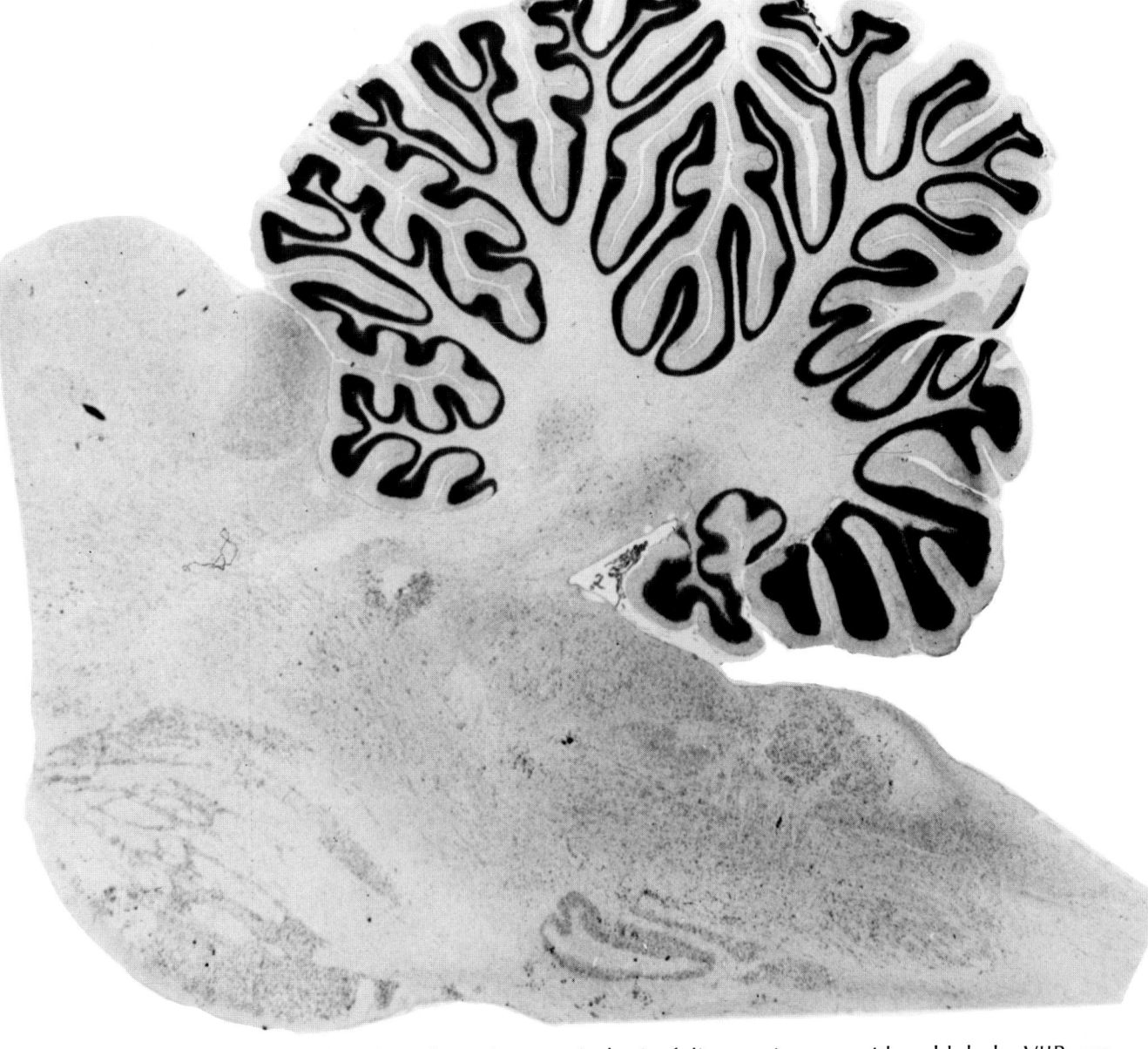

Figs. 19–20 This section is taken lateral to Figures 17–18. The paramedian lobule (Larsell's copular and posterior parts) is prominent, and its continuity with the medullary core at the base of sublobules VIIIA and VIIIB is apparent when compared with Figures 15–16. Also of interest is the beginning of the parafloccular peduncle, issuing from the medullary core at the base of vermal lobule IX and caudal VIIIB. The nodulus (**lobule X**) extends further laterally than any other vermal structure. The hem-

ispheric folia continuous with sublobule VIIB are identified as the pars anterior of the paramedian lobule (**PAP**), as described in the Introduction (see p. 11).

The fastigial nucleus (**FN**) is reduced in size, and both the anterior (**AIN**) and posterior (**PIN**) interposed nuclei have appeared. The superior cerebellar peduncle is prominent, while only a vestige of vermal folium I$_c$ is present.   *Nissl. X 8.*

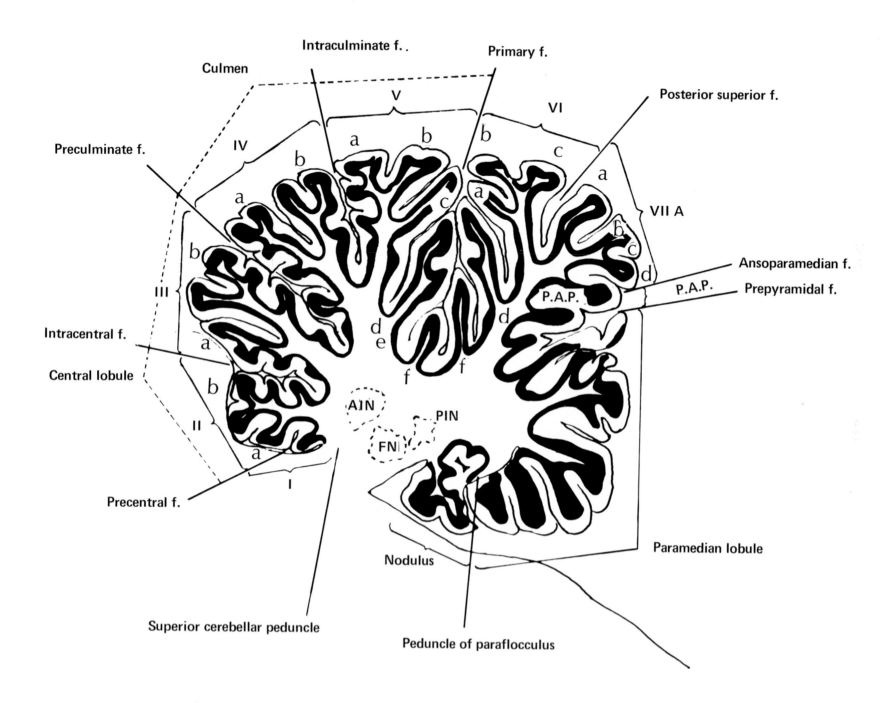

Culmen

Intraculminate f. .

Primary f.

Preculminate f.

Posterior superior f.

IV

V

VI

b

a

b

b

c

a

b

c

a

VII A

a

III

c

a

b

c

b

Intracentral f.

d

P.A.P.

Ansoparamedian f.

Central lobule

a

d

e

P.A.P.

Prepyramidal f.

b

e

f

f

II

AIN

PIN

f

a

FN

Precentral f.

I

Paramedian lobule

Nodulus

Superior cerebellar peduncle

Peduncle of paraflocculus

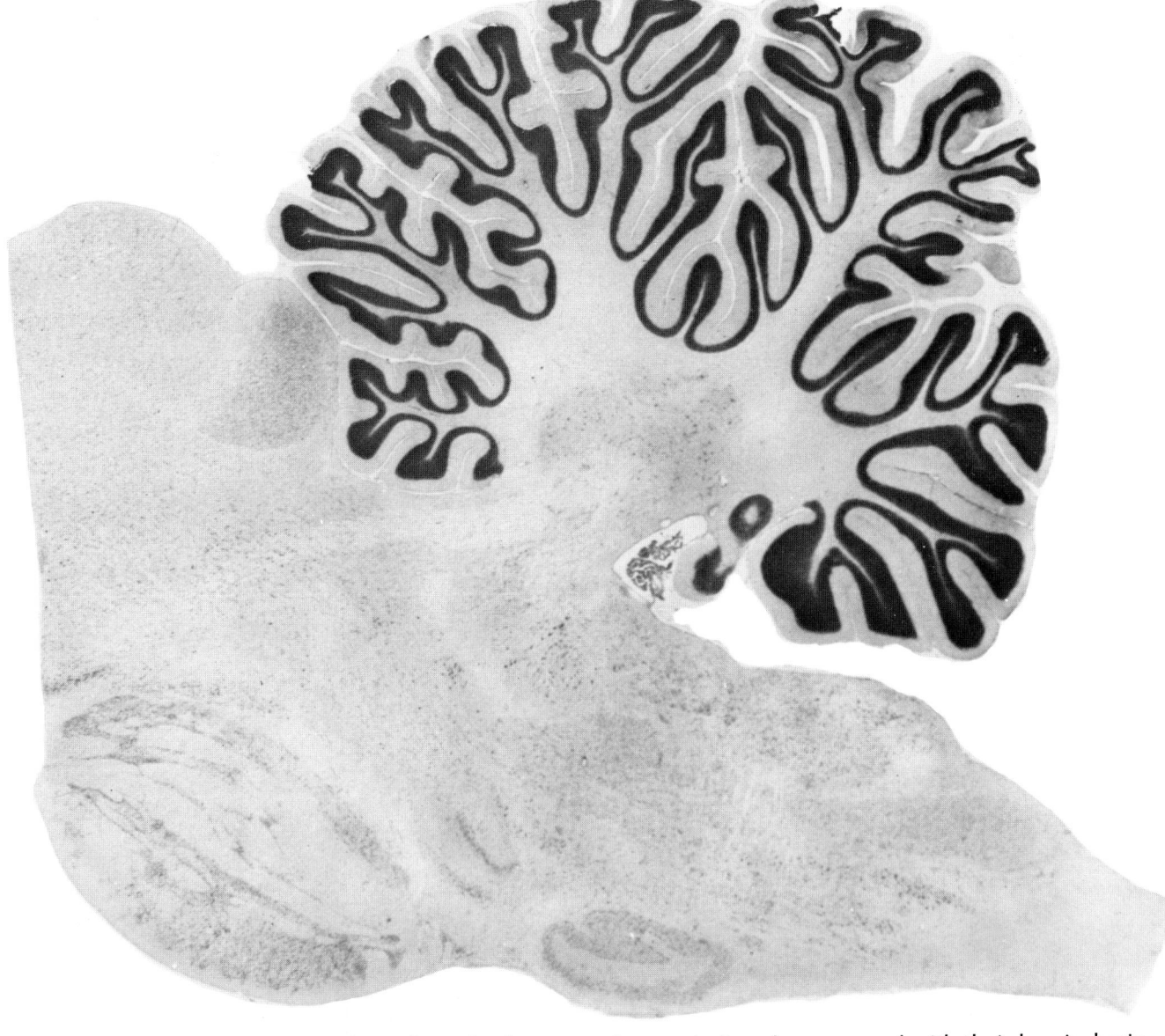

Figs. 21–22 This section is taken through the medial part of the cerebellar hemisphere. The parafloccular peduncle and the paramedian lobule are prominent, and are in positions similar to those of Figures 19–20. The nodulus (**lobule X**) has decreased in size, and only its medullary base is noticeable. The pars anterior of the paramedian lobule (**PAP**) appears in its previous position, while only a vestige of the lingula remains. Vermal lobules of the anterior cerebellum have merged with their hemispheric counterparts: lobules II and III forming the central lobule, and lobules IV and V (**culmen**) forming the anterior quadrangular lobule.

The anterior (**AIN**) and posterior (**PIN**) interposed nuclei are prominent, and the posterior superior fissure still lies between lobule VI and sublobule VIIA. *Nissl. X 8.*

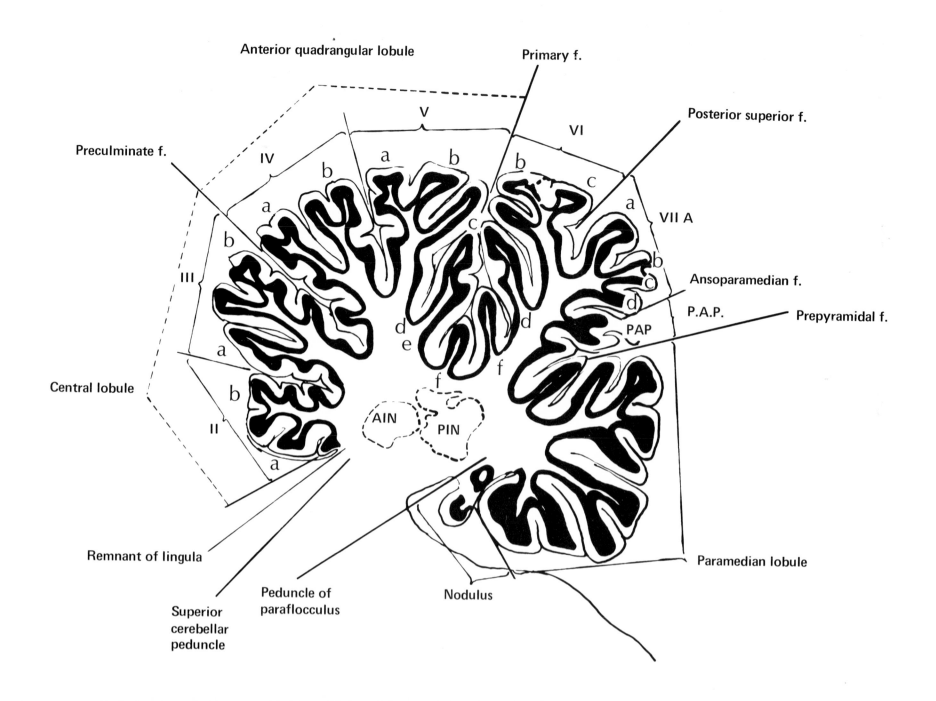

Anterior quadrangular lobule

Primary f.

Posterior superior f.

Preculminate f.

Ansoparamedian f.

P.A.P.

Prepyramidal f.

Central lobule

Remnant of lingula

Superior
cerebellar
peduncle

Peduncle of
paraflocculus

Nodulus

Paramedian lobule

III

IV

V

VI

VII A

II

AIN

PIN

PAP

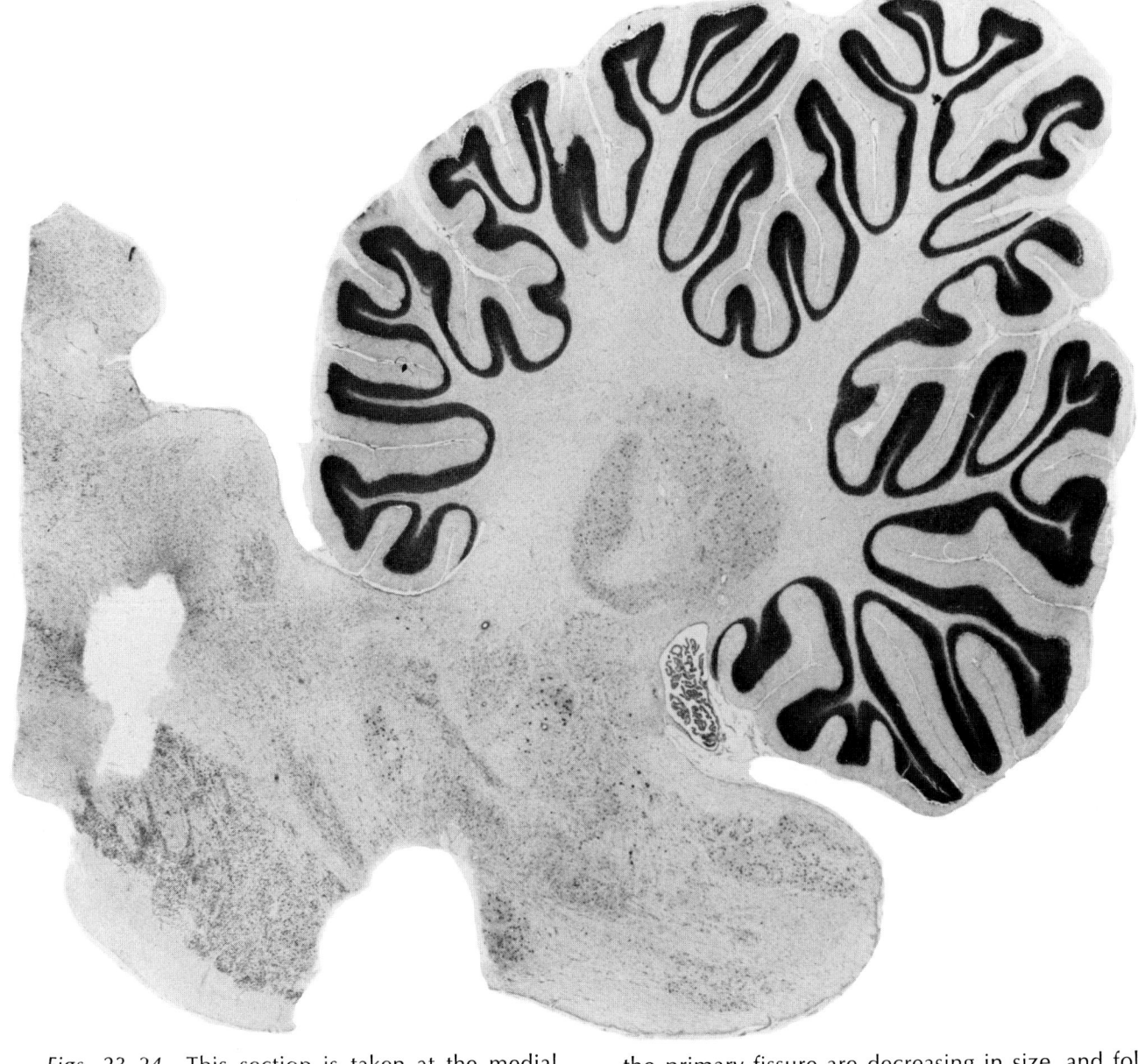

Figs. 23–24 This section is taken at the medial border of the simple lobule. Folium VIIA$_a$ can be seen extending anteriorly to form the posterior part of the simple lobule. The posterior superior fissure, which further laterally will delimit the simple lobule from crus I and II (see p. 10 and Figures 25–26), now lies caudal to folium VIIA$_a$, Folia VIIA$_{b,c,d}$ are less distinct, and are merging laterally with a medullary core which will give rise to the ansiform lobule (**crus I** and **II**). The pars anterior of the paramedian lobule (**PAP**) is reduced in size, and lies buried in the depths of the prepyramidal fissure. The folia in the primary fissure are decreasing in size, and folia V$_d$ and V$_e$ have merged.

The paramedian lobule is enormous in this plane, and the first folium of the dorsal paraflocculus can be seen emanating from the peduncle of the paraflocculus. These folia have been numbered in order to maintain continuity from one section to the next. Folium 1 is the most caudomedial, and folium 10 is the most rostrolateral. The position of the peduncle of the flocculus is noted, although its silhouette is obscured.   *Nissl. X 8.*

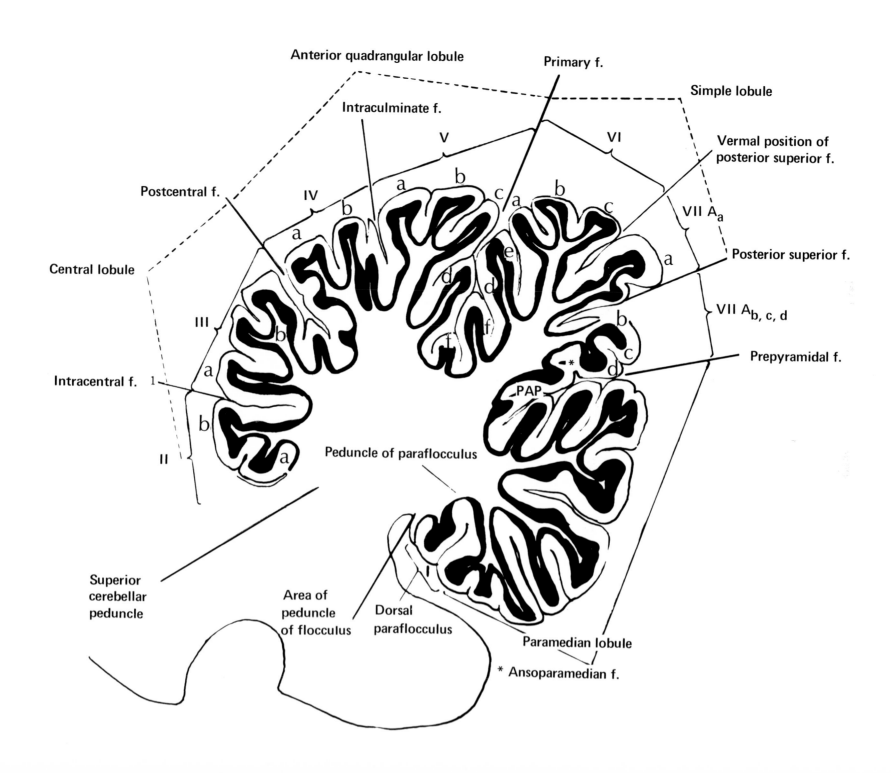

Anterior quadrangular lobule

Primary f.

Intraculminate f.

Simple lobule

Vermal position of posterior superior f.

Postcentral f.

Central lobule

Posterior superior f.

Intracentral f.

Peduncle of paraflocculus

Superior cerebellar peduncle

Area of peduncle of flocculus

Dorsal paraflocculus

Paramedian lobule

* Ansoparamedian f.

Prepyramidal f.

PAP

VII A$_a$

VII A$_{b, c, d}$

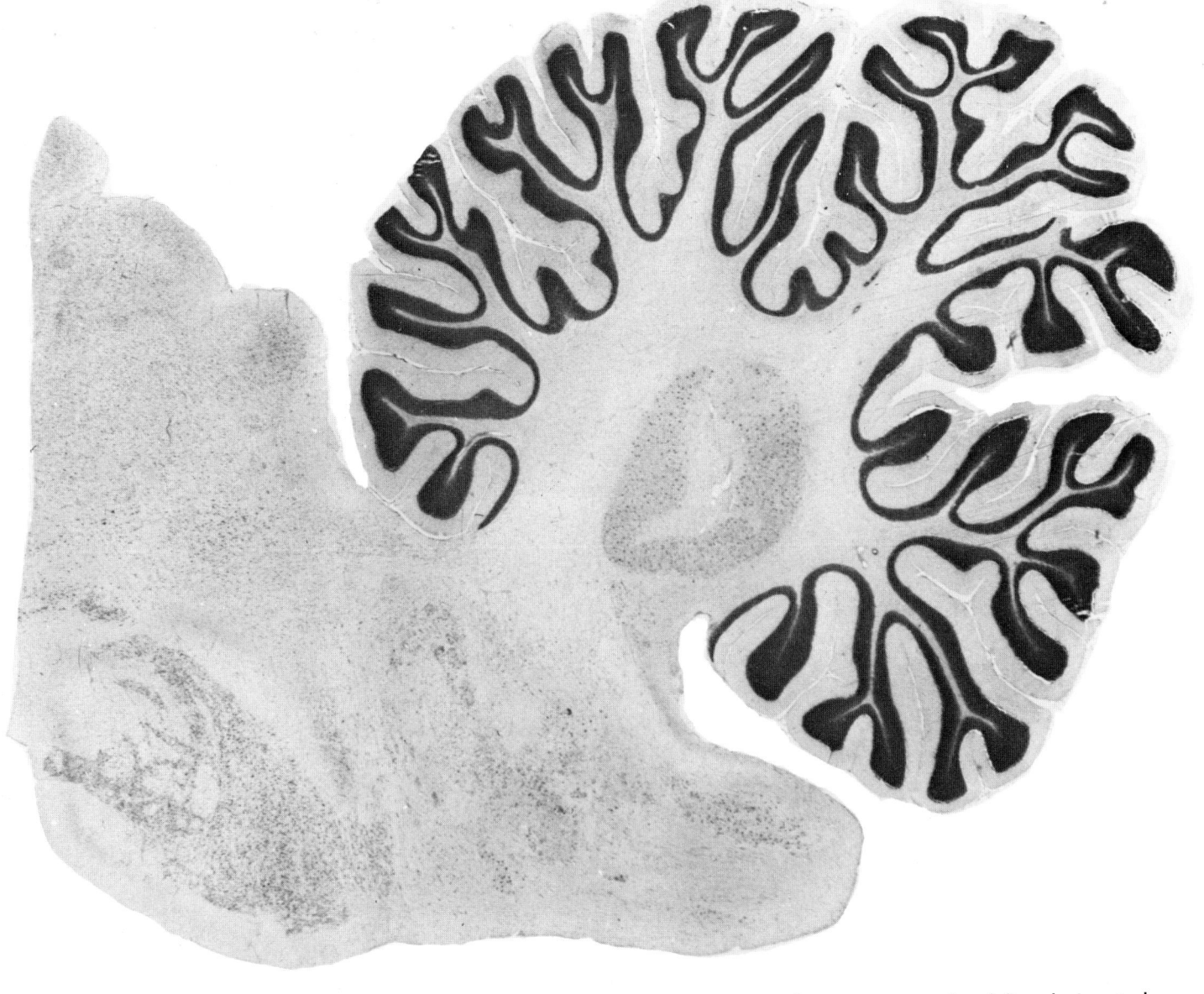

Figs. 25–26   The ansiform lobule has a medullary core continuous with vermal VIIA$_{b,c,d}$. At this level crus II$_p$ is most prominent, but in successive sections crus II$_a$, I$_p$, and I$_a$ will be seen emerging from this same medullary core.

The simple lobule is more distinct, with a single medullary core. Its three anterior folia, designated by letters **a**, **b**, and **c**, are derived from vermal lobule VI, and its two posterior folia, designated **a** and **a′**, are derived from the single vermal folium VIIA$_a$.

The dentate nucleus (**DN**) is seen clearly in this plane, and is quite large, while the interposed nuclei are absent. The small vestibulocerebellar nucleus (**VC**) can be seen ventral to the dentate nucleus. *Nissl. X 8.*

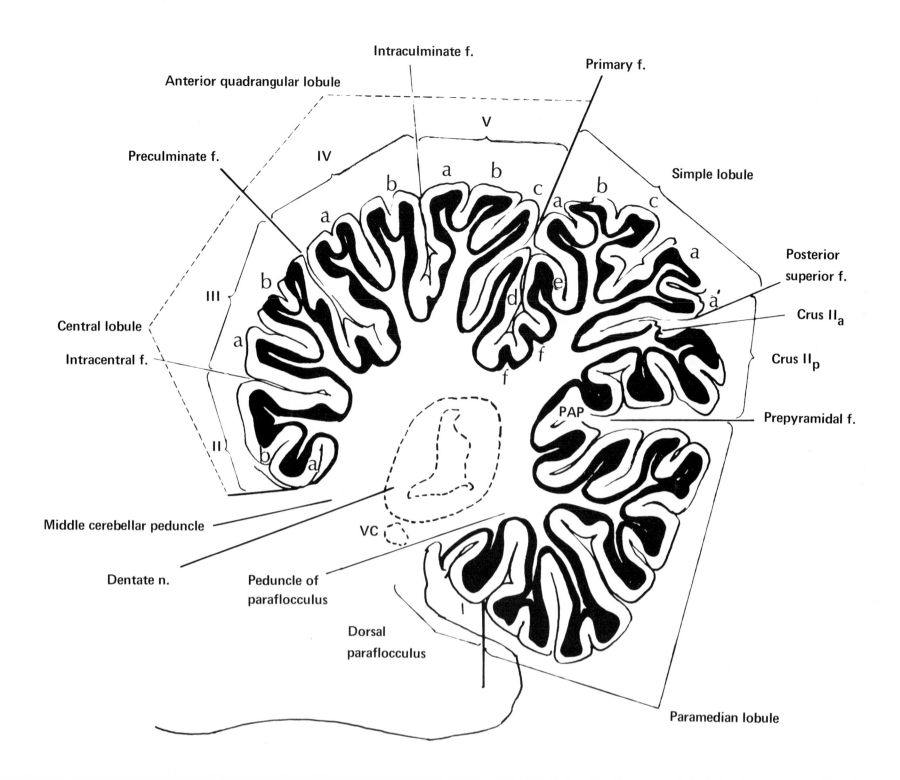

Intraculminate f.

Primary f.

Anterior quadrangular lobule

V

Preculminate f.

IV

Simple lobule

b

a

b

c

a

b

c

a

a

a

a'

Posterior superior f.

b

III

Crus II$_a$

Central lobule

a

d

e

Crus II$_p$

Intracentral f.

f

f

II

f

b

a

PAP

Prepyramidal f.

Middle cerebellar peduncle

VC

Dentate n.

Peduncle of paraflocculus

Dorsal paraflocculus

Paramedian lobule

41

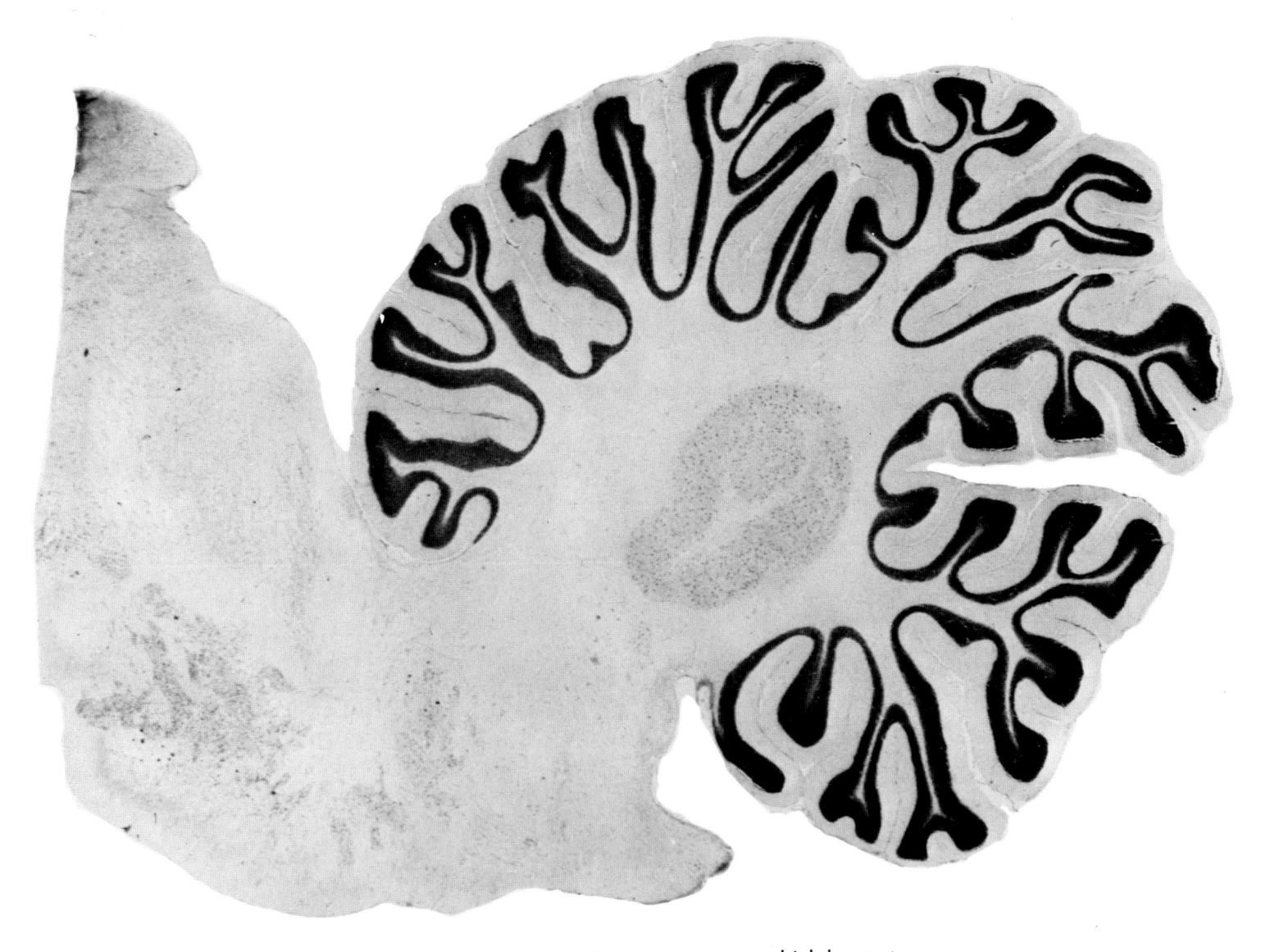

Figs. 27–28 In this section crus II$_a$, which has not yet reached the surface, emerges from the medullary core of the ansiform lobule, anteriorly to crus II$_p$. The second folium of the dorsal paraflocculus is evident and the paramedian lobule is prominent.

The simple lobule, with its five surface folia and prominent medullary core, is unchanged.   *Nissl.* X 8.

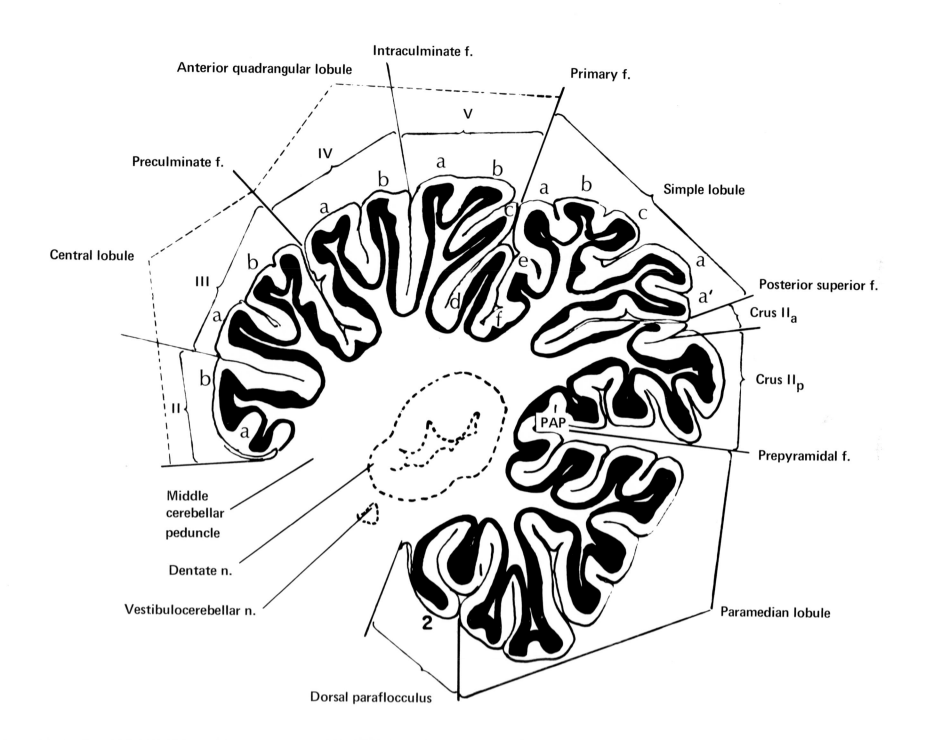

Intraculminate f.

Anterior quadrangular lobule

Primary f.

V

IV

b a b

Preculminate f.

b a b

a c

Simple lobule

a

Central lobule

III

b

e

c

Posterior superior f.

a

d f

a

a'

Crus II_a

II

b

Crus II_p

a

PAP

Prepyramidal f.

Middle
cerebellar
peduncle

Dentate n.

Vestibulocerebellar n.

2

Paramedian lobule

Dorsal paraflocculus

43

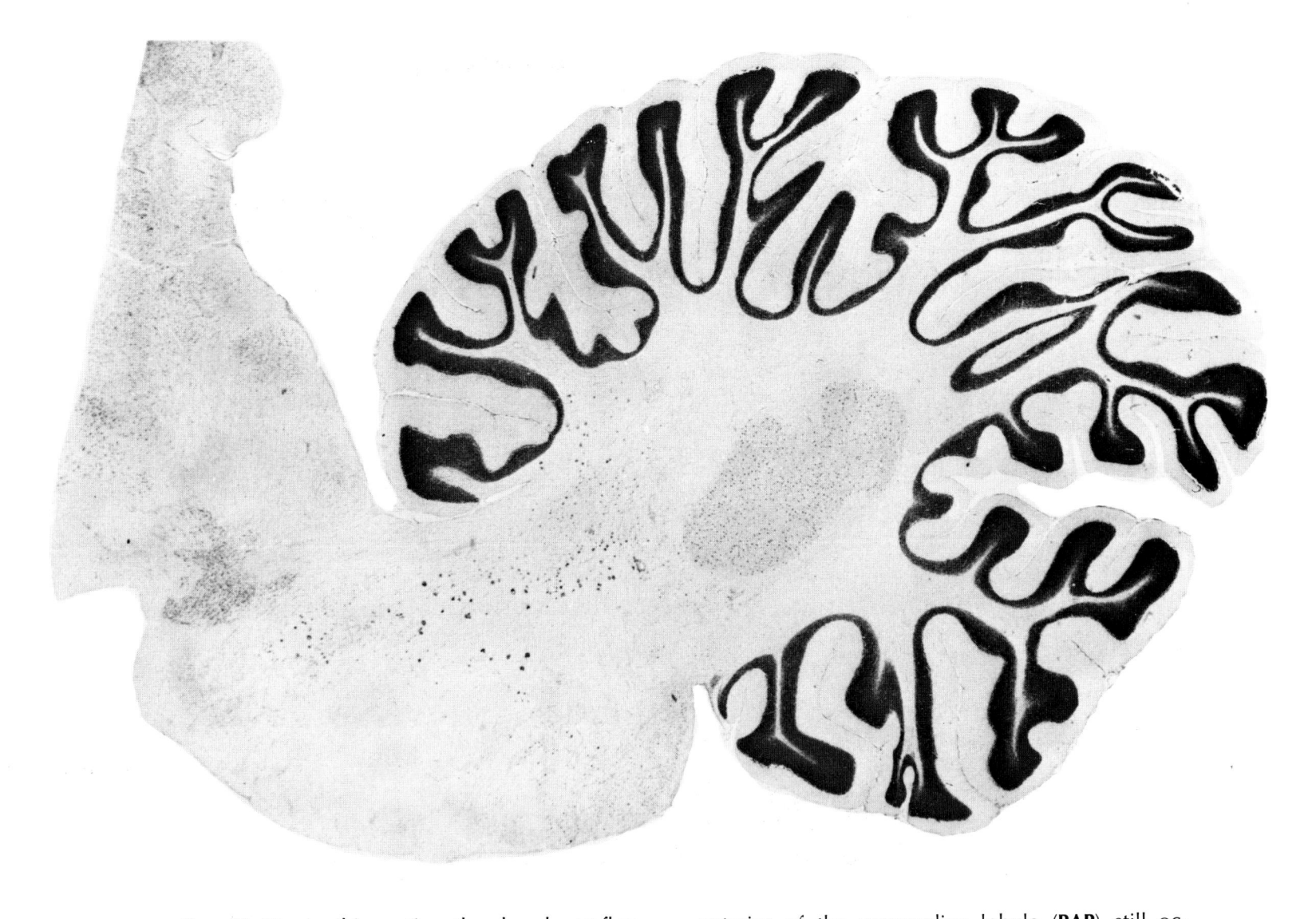

Figs. 29–30 In this section the dorsal parafloc-culus has developed a third folium. Crus II_p and II_a are seen, and the medullary core of crus I separates anteriorly from the core of the ansiform lobule in the depths of the posterior superior fissure. The middle cerebellar peduncle is prominent and the paramedian lobule is decreasing in size. The pars anterior of the paramedian lobule (**PAP**) still oc-cupies the depths of the prepyramidal fissure.

The simple lobule is unchanged and the primary fissure now contains only folia VI_d, VI_e, and V_c. The central lobule, anterior quadrangular lobule, vesti-bulocerebellar nucleus, and dentate nucleus remain unchanged. *Nissl. X 8.*

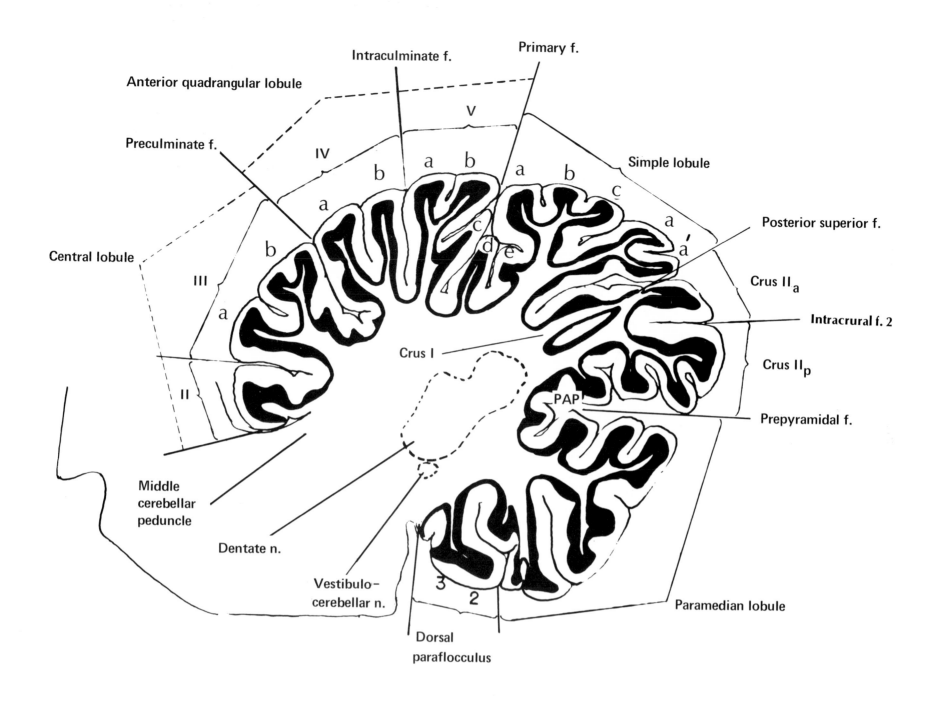

Anterior quadrangular lobule

Intraculminate f.

Primary f.

Preculminate f.

Simple lobule

Posterior superior f.

Central lobule

Crus II~a~

Intracrural f. 2

Crus I

Crus II~p~

PAP

Prepyramidal f.

Middle cerebellar peduncle

Dentate n.

Vestibulo-cerebellar n.

Paramedian lobule

Dorsal paraflocculus

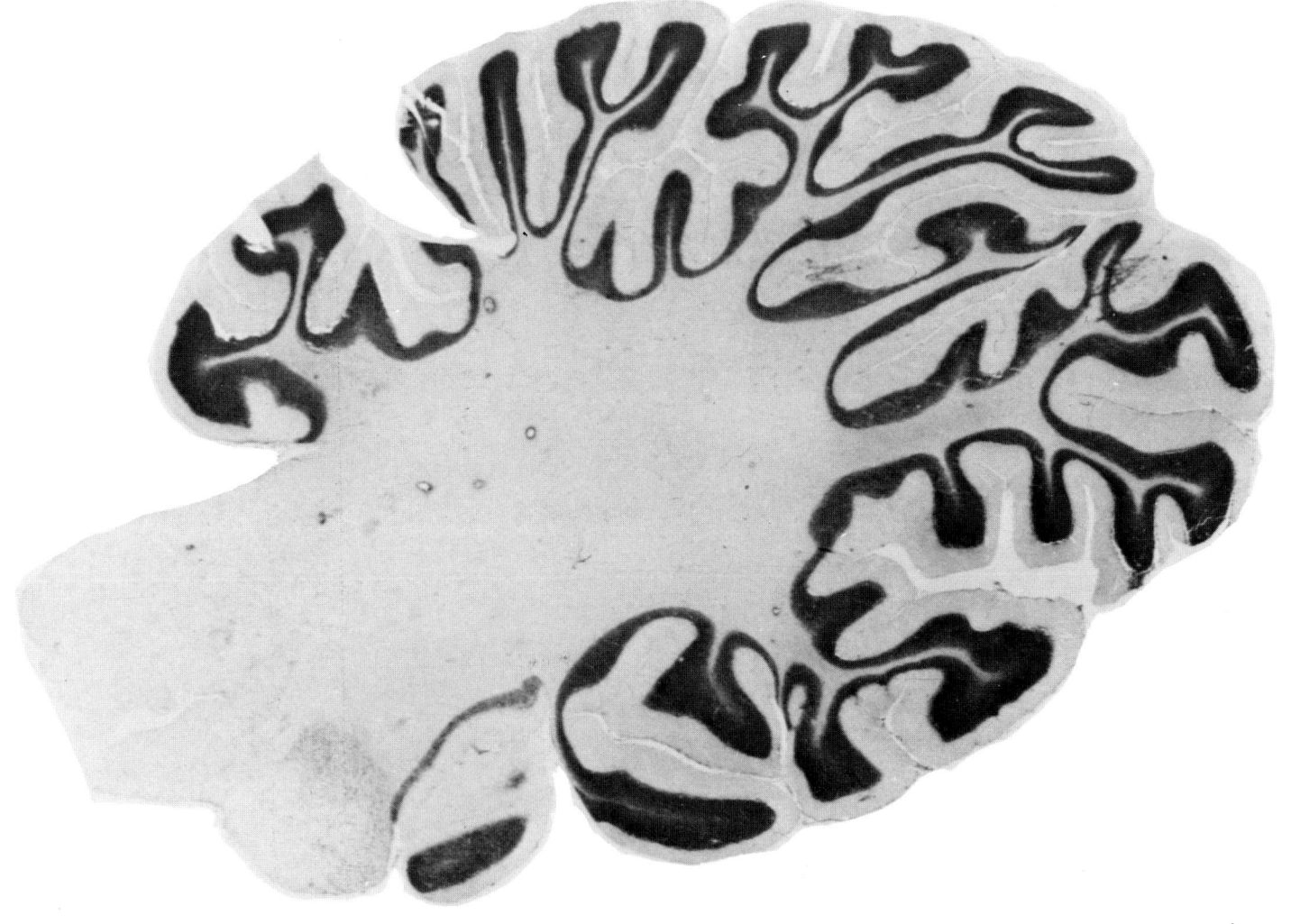

Figs. 31–32 In this section, the central lobule is reduced in size, with only two surface folia remaining. The simple lobule now exhibits only four distinct surface folia: folia **b** and **c** (derived from lobule VI) have merged.

Crus I has not yet reached the surface, but both crus II$_a$ and II$_p$ are prominent. Only a vestige of the paramedian lobule remains, and the fourth folium of the dorsal paraflocculus has emerged.

The most medial folium of the flocculus is seen in this section. The lobulation of this portion of the the floccular folia is less definitive than that for the paraflocculus and is presented mainly for orienta-

tion in moving from one section to another. According to Larsell (1953), the flocculus has eleven folia. Only ten could be counted in our serial sections, and they are numbered accordingly.

The pars anterior of the paramedian lobule (**PAP**) is still represented by a single folium in the depths of the prepyramidal fissure. Note that the posterolateral fissure, which separates lobule X from lobule IX in the vermis, may now be seen in the hemisphere separating the flocculus (related to vermal lobule X) from the paraflocculus (related to vermal lobule IX). *Nissl. X 10.*

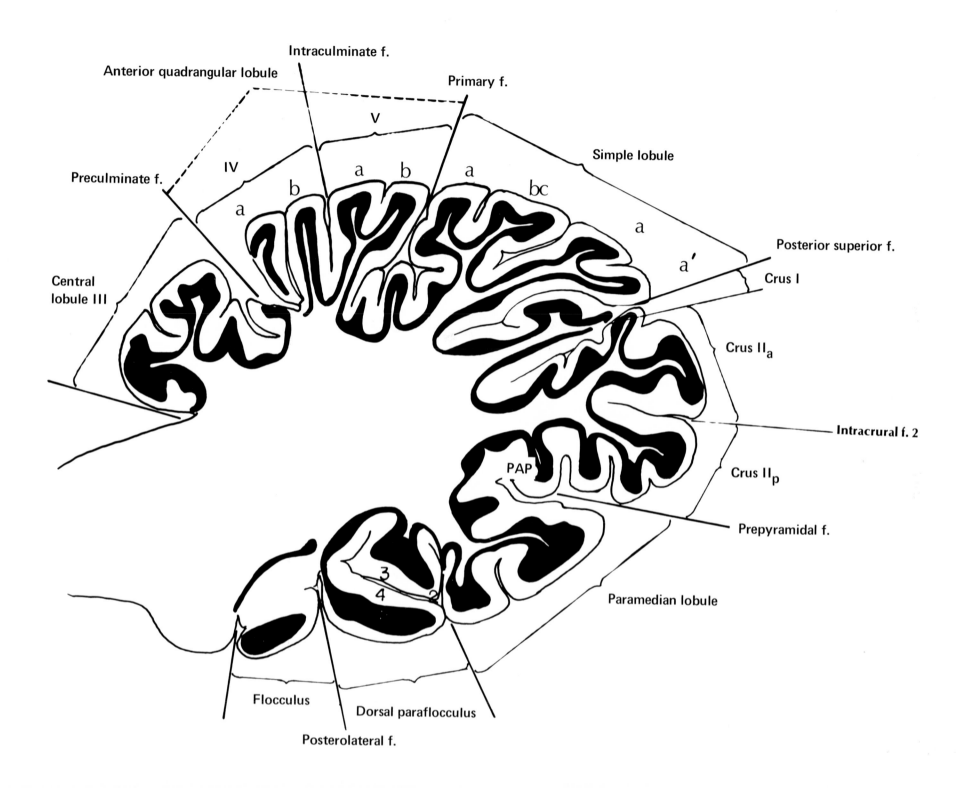

Intraculminate f.

Anterior quadrangular lobule

Primary f.

V

Simple lobule

Preculminate f.

IV

b

a

b

a

bc

a

Central
lobule III

a

a'

Posterior superior f.

Crus I

Crus II_a

Intracrural f. 2

PAP

Crus II_p

Prepyramidal f.

3
4

Paramedian lobule

Flocculus

Dorsal paraflocculus

Posterolateral f.

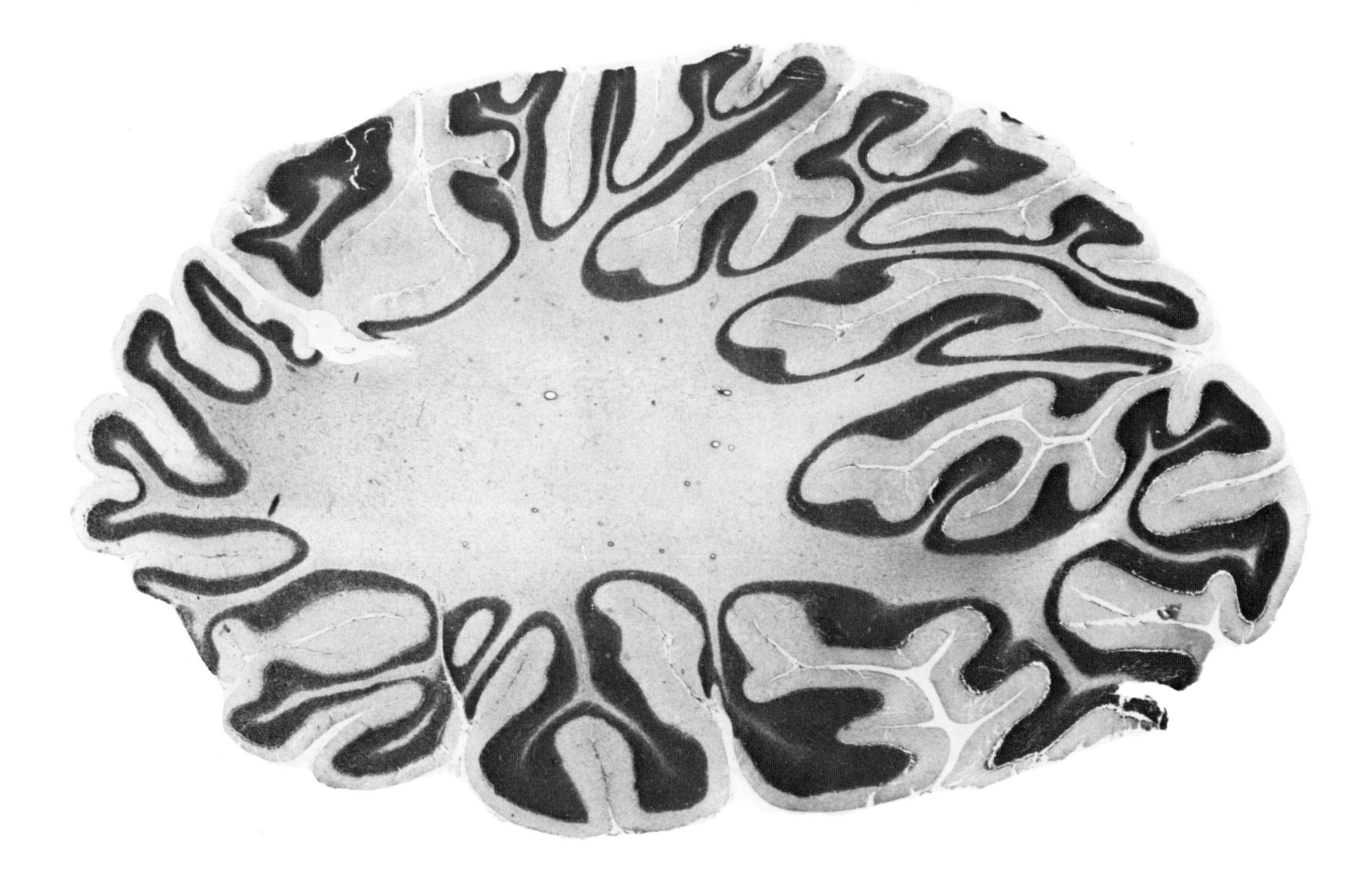

Figs. 33–34 In this section the superior cerebellar peduncle has disappeared and the cerebellar hemisphere is free of the brain stem. Crus I has reached the surface, and crus II$_a$ and II$_p$ are prominent. Only a vestige of the paramedian lobule remains, and only a trace of the pars anterior of the paramedian lobule (**PAP**) can be seen.

Folia 4 and 5 of the dorsal paraflocculus have appeared, and most of the ten folia of the flocculus can be seen emerging from the central medullary substance of the cerebellar hemisphere.

Only a small part of the central lobule is present, and the anterior quadrangular lobule is reduced in size. Folium V$_c$ lies in the depths of the primary fissure. The four folia of the simple lobule are distinct, while the anterior portion of the cerebellum has become smaller.   *Nissl. X 10.*

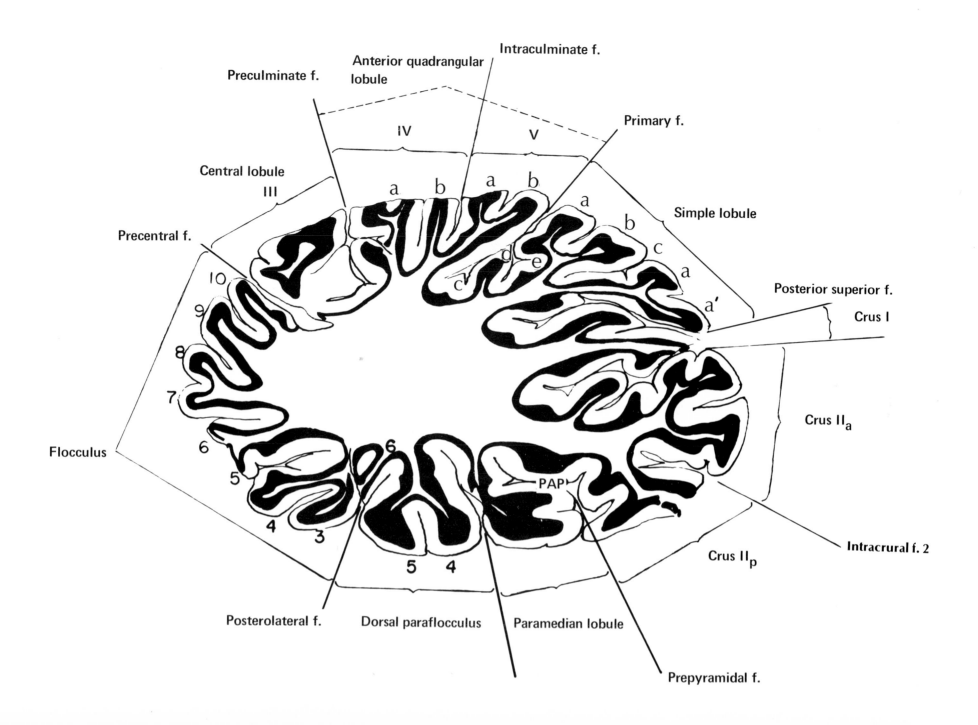

Preculminate f.

Anterior quadrangular
lobule

Intraculminate f.

Primary f.

Central lobule
III

IV

a   b   a   b

V

a

Simple lobule

b

c

a

Precentral f.

c

d
e

a'

Posterior superior f.

10

Crus I

9

8

7

Crus II_a

6

Flocculus

5

6

6

4

3

PAP

5   4

Crus II_p

Intracrural f. 2

Posterolateral f.

Dorsal paraflocculus

Paramedian lobule

Prepyramidal f.

49

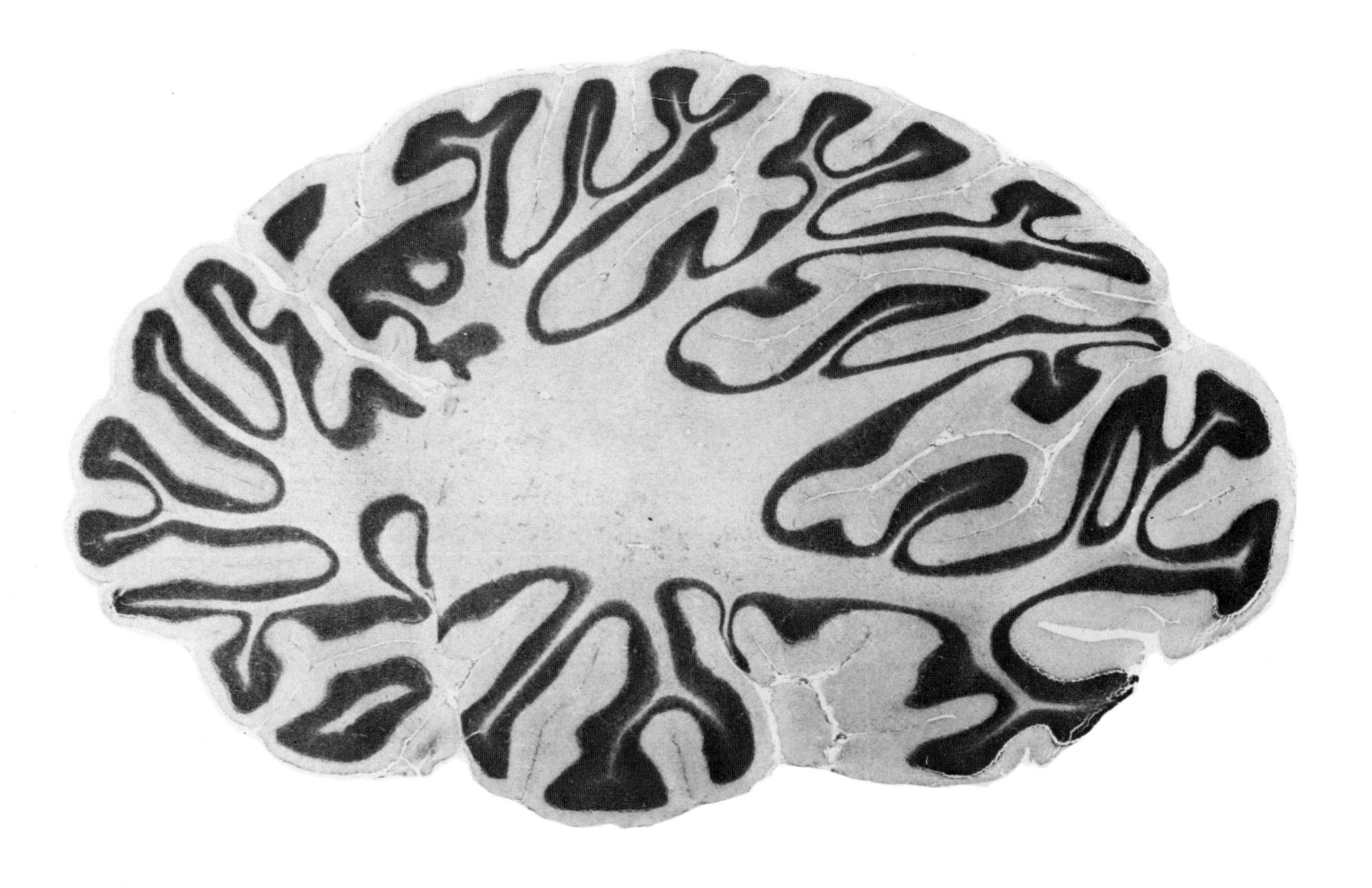

Figs. 35–36 In this section folia 4, 5, and 6 of
the dorsal paraflocculus are seen, as are folia 3
through 10 of the flocculus. Crus II_a and II_p occupy
most of the posterior surface of the hemisphere,
and the simple lobule is a prominent structure on
the dorsal surface. The anterior quadrangle lobule is
distinct at this level, but the central lobule has disappeared. A trace of the paramedian lobule (**PL**)
remains.   *Nissl. X 10.*

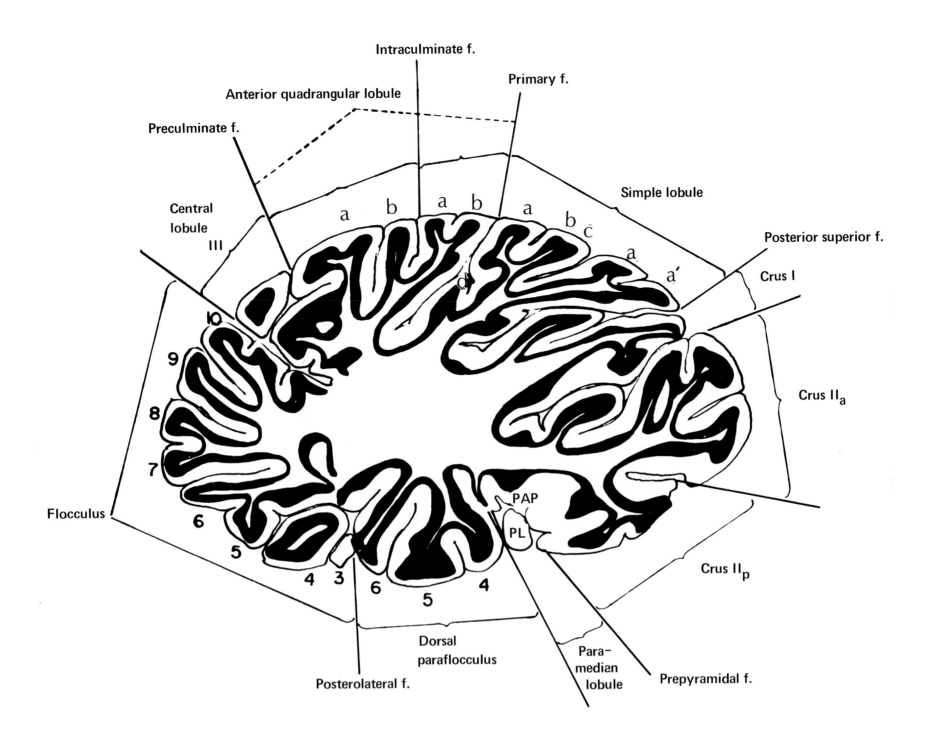

Intraculminate f.

Primary f.

Anterior quadrangular lobule

Preculminate f.

Simple lobule

Central
lobule

III

a   b   a   b   a   b   c̄

a

a'

Posterior superior f.

Crus I

Crus II_a

10

9

8

7

Flocculus

6

5

4   3

6

5

4

PAP

PL

Crus II_p

Dorsal
paraflocculus

Para-
median
lobule

Prepyramidal f.

Posterolateral f.

51

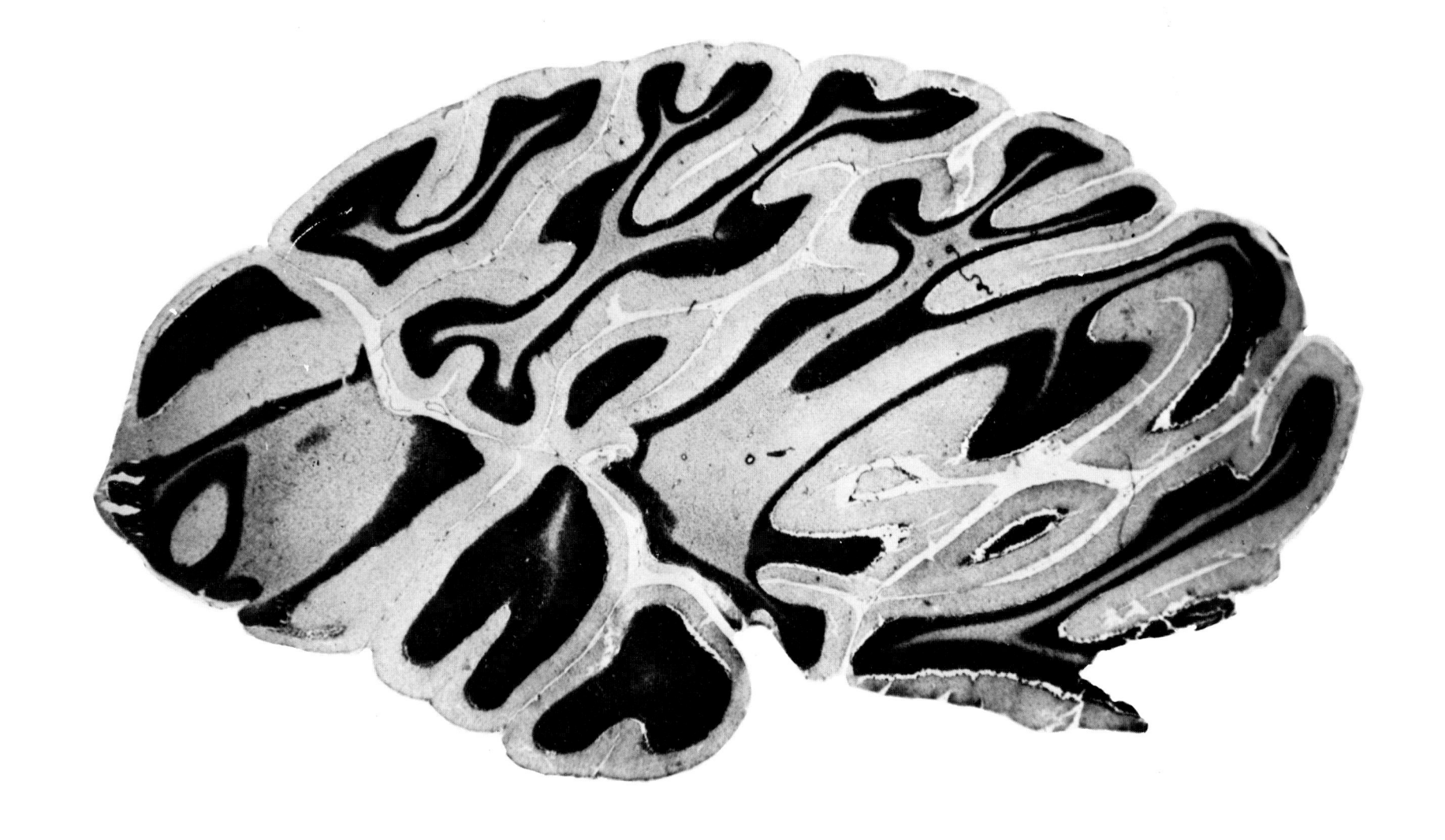

Figs. 39–40 Crus II$_p$ has entirely disappeared, and crus II$_a$ is now smaller than crus I$_a$ and I$_p$, which have become the largest lobules in this section. The flocculus is no longer present, and the most distal folia of the dorsal paraflocculus (6 through 10) are present. The simple lobule and anterior quadrangular lobule remain anteriorly.   *Nissl. X 12.*

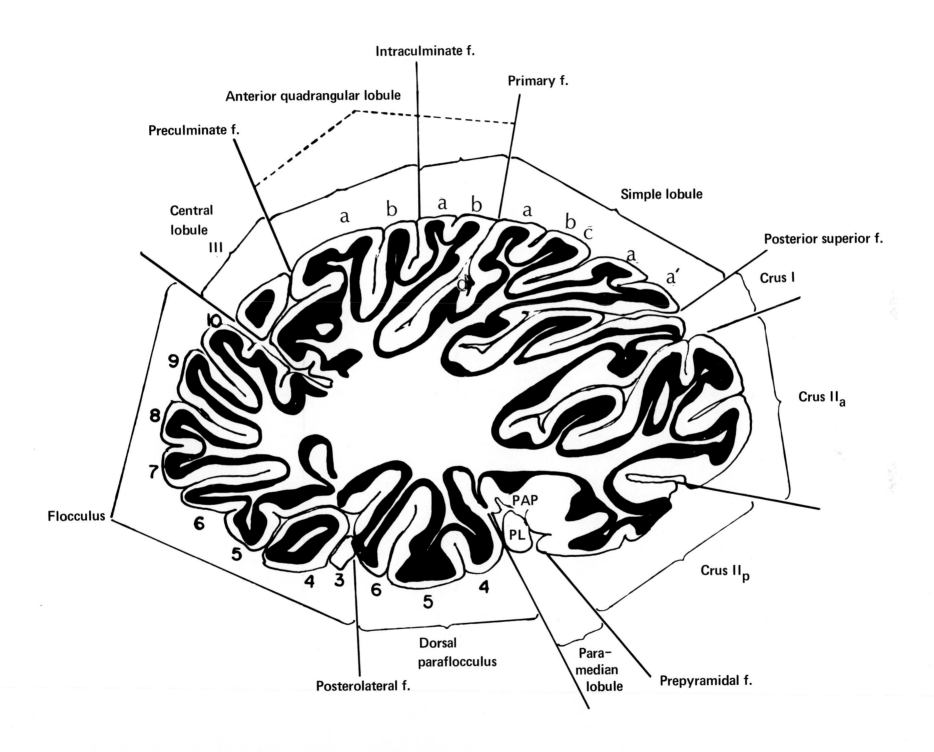

Intraculminate f.

Anterior quadrangular lobule

Primary f.

Preculminate f.

Simple lobule

Central
lobule
III

a b a b a b c

a

a'

Posterior superior f.

Crus I

10

Crus II_a

9

8

7

Flocculus

6

5

PAP

PL

Crus II_p

4 3

6

5

4

Dorsal
paraflocculus

Para-
median
lobule

Posterolateral f.

Prepyramidal f.

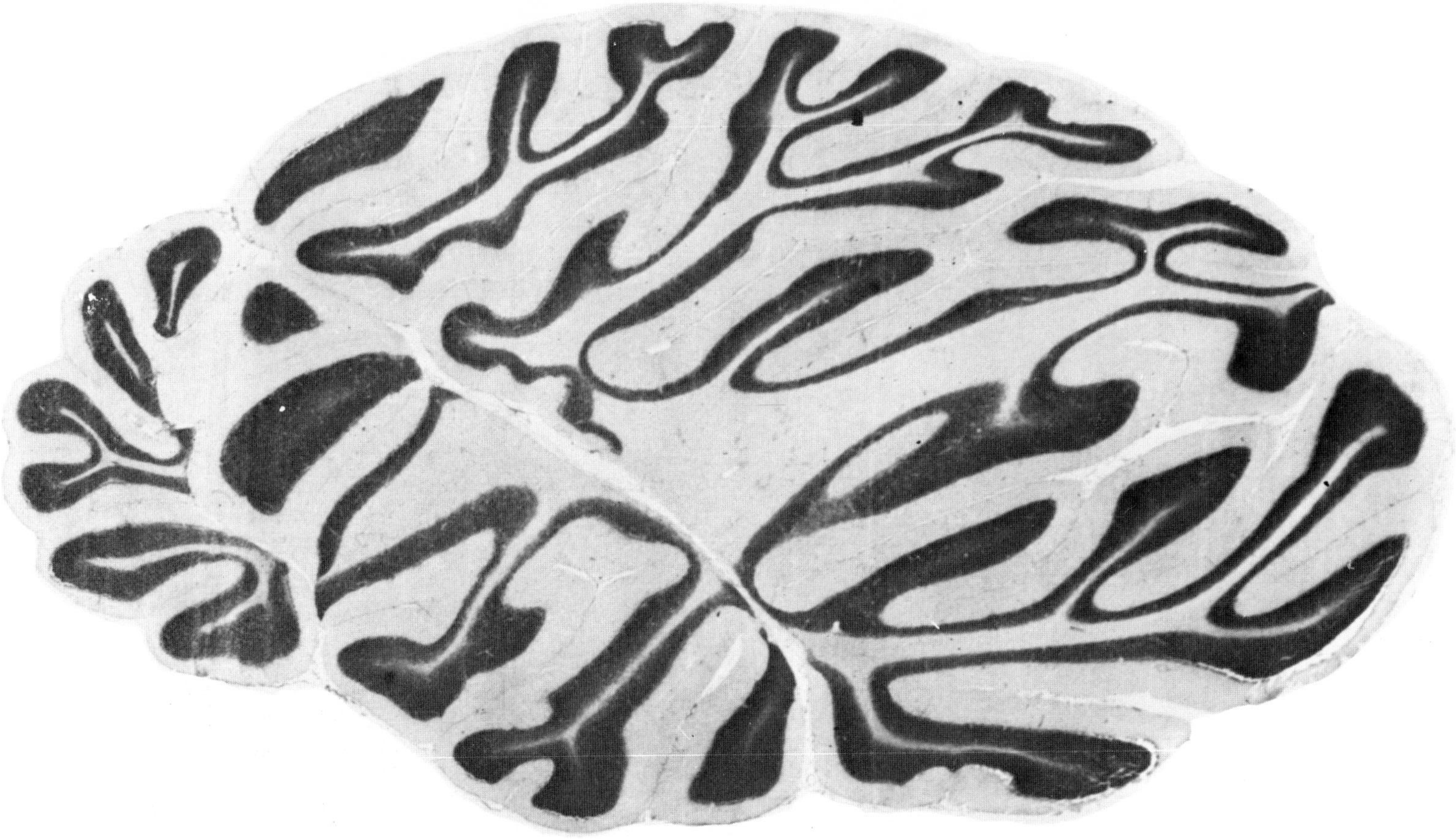

Figs. 37–38 The cerebellar medullary core common to the hemisphere, paraflocculus, and flocculus has disappeared, and these structures are now clearly separated. The anterior quadrangular lobule and simple lobule are still prominent. Crus I_a and I_p are as large as crus II_a, but crus II_p is reduced in size. *Nissl. X 11.*

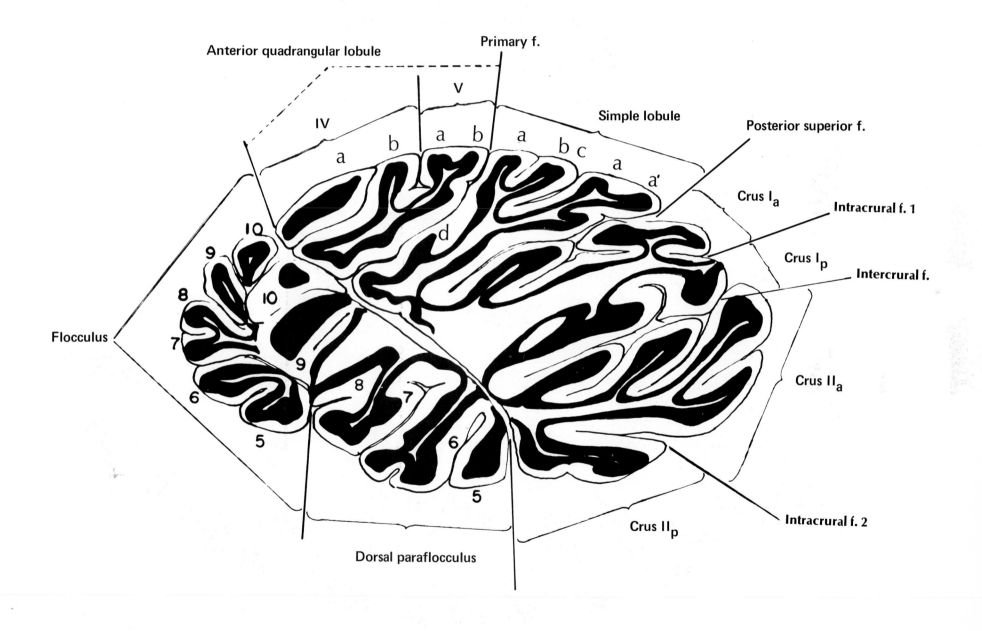

Anterior quadrangular lobule

Primary f.

V

IV

Simple lobule

a   b   a   b   a   b   c   a

a

d

a'

Posterior superior f.

Crus I_a

Intracrural f. 1

Crus I_p

Intercrural f.

10

9

8

10

7

9

8

7

6

6

5

5

Crus II_a

Flocculus

Dorsal paraflocculus

Crus II_p

Intracrural f. 2

53

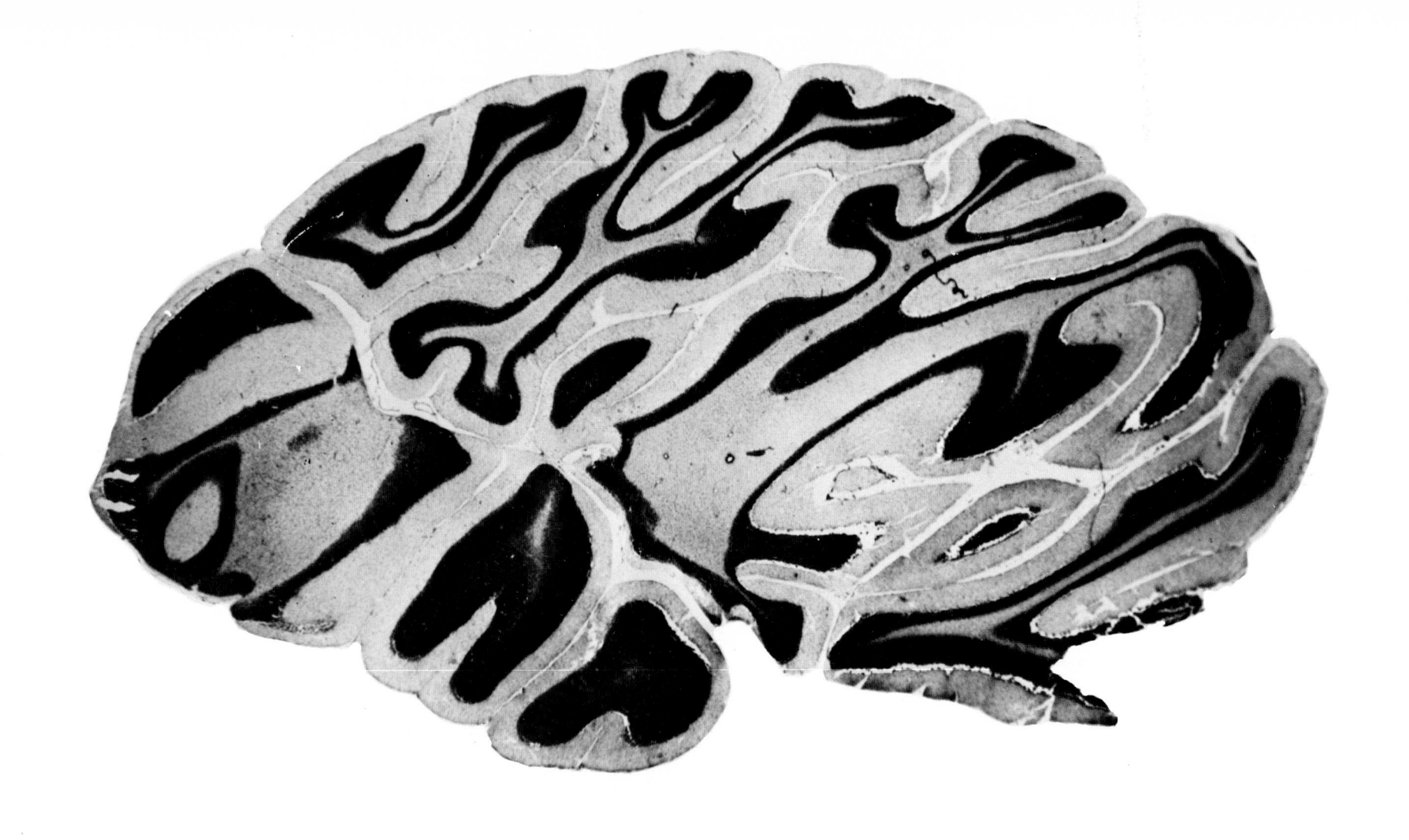

Figs. 39–40 Crus II_p has entirely disappeared, and crus II_a is now smaller than crus I_a and I_p, which have become the largest lobules in this section. The flocculus is no longer present, and the most distal folia of the dorsal paraflocculus (6 through 10) are present. The simple lobule and anterior quadrangular lobule remain anteriorly.   *Nissl. X 12.*

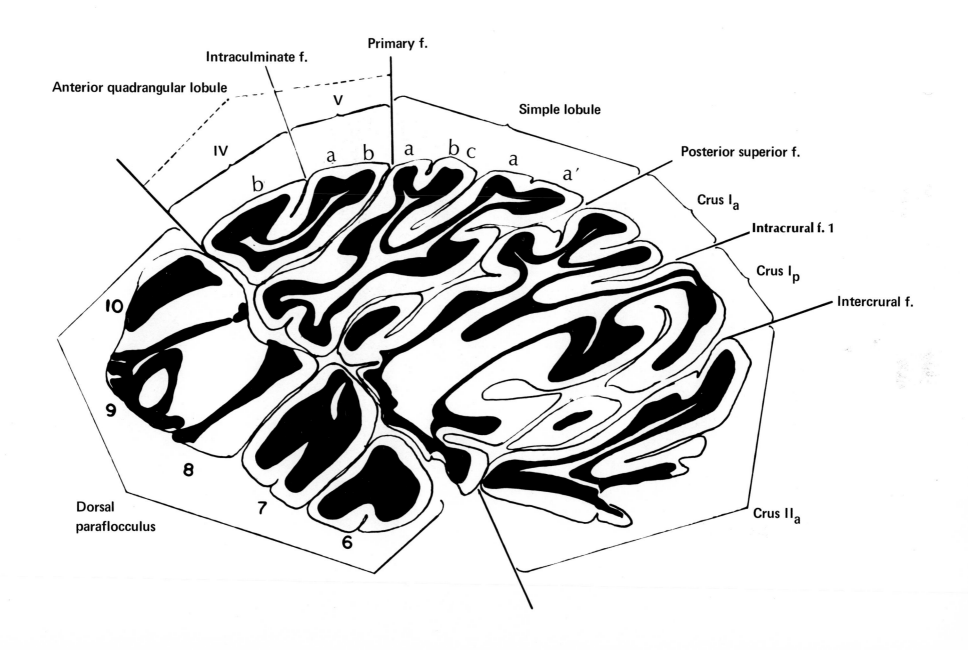

Intraculminate f.

Primary f.

Anterior quadrangular lobule

V

Simple lobule

IV

a b a b c a a′

b

Posterior superior f.

Crus I$_a$

Intracrural f. 1

Crus I$_p$

Intercrural f.

10

9

8

7

6

Dorsal paraflocculus

Crus II$_a$

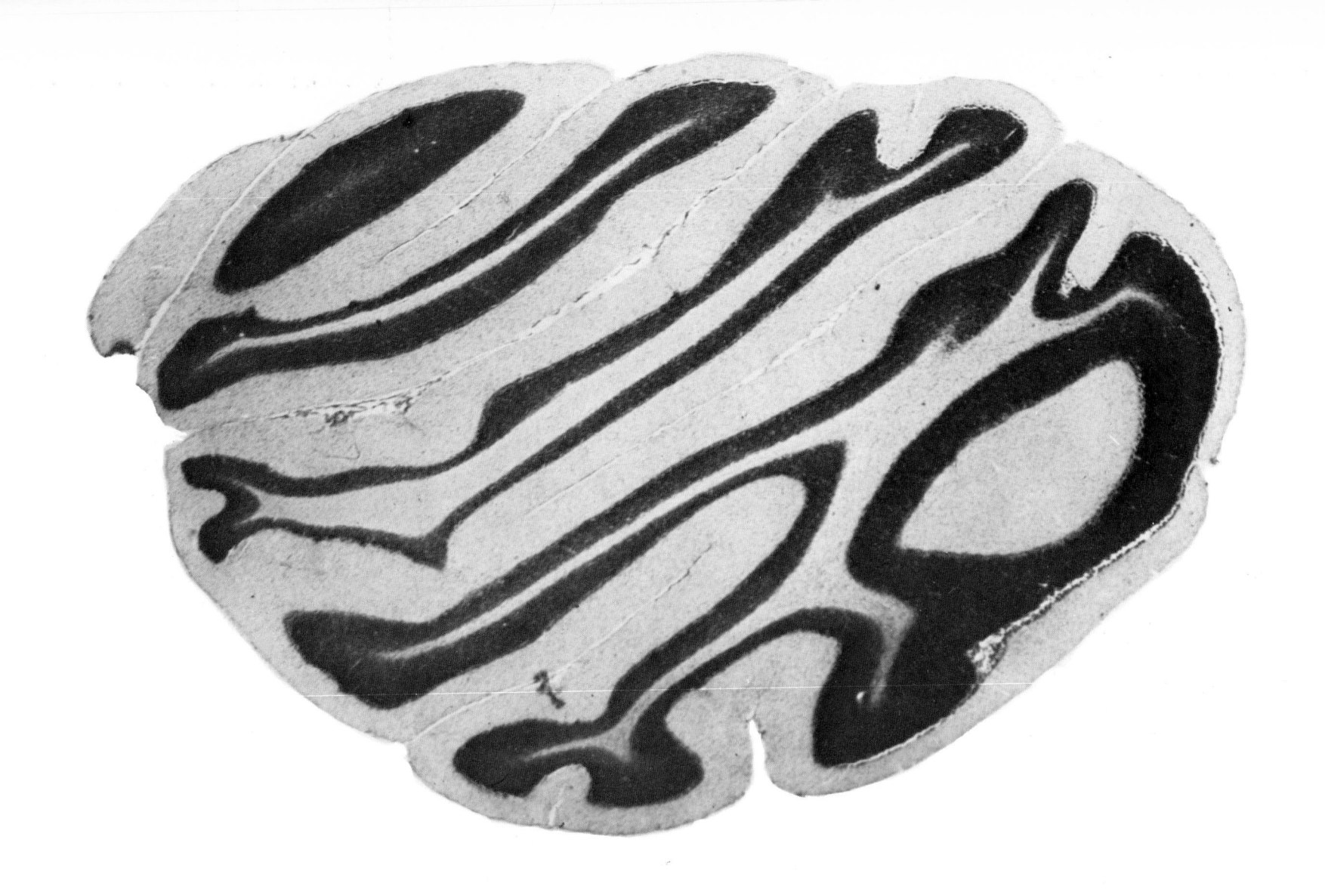

Figs. 41–42 The prominence of crus I$_p$ and I$_a$ is striking in this most lateral section through the hemispheres. The anterior quadrangular and simple lobules extend to this lateral region, and both these lobules and crus I$_a$ and I$_p$ reach the inferior surface of the hemisphere   *Nissl. X 17.*

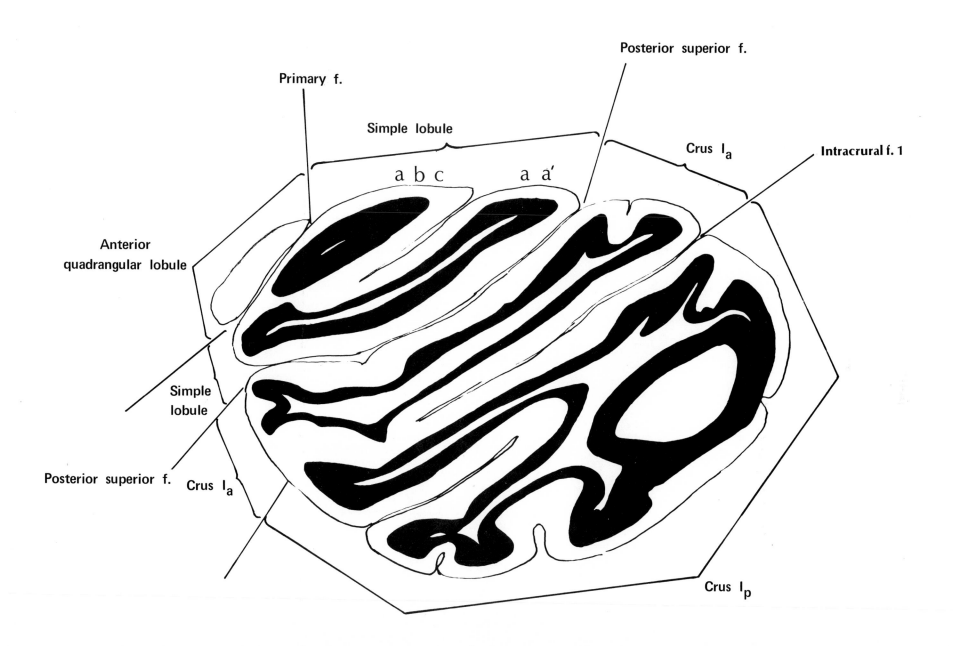

Primary f.

Posterior superior f.

Simple lobule

Crus I$_a$

Intracrural f. 1

a b c   a a'

Anterior
quadrangular lobule

Simple
lobule

Posterior superior f.   Crus I$_a$

Crus I$_p$

Horizontal Section Series

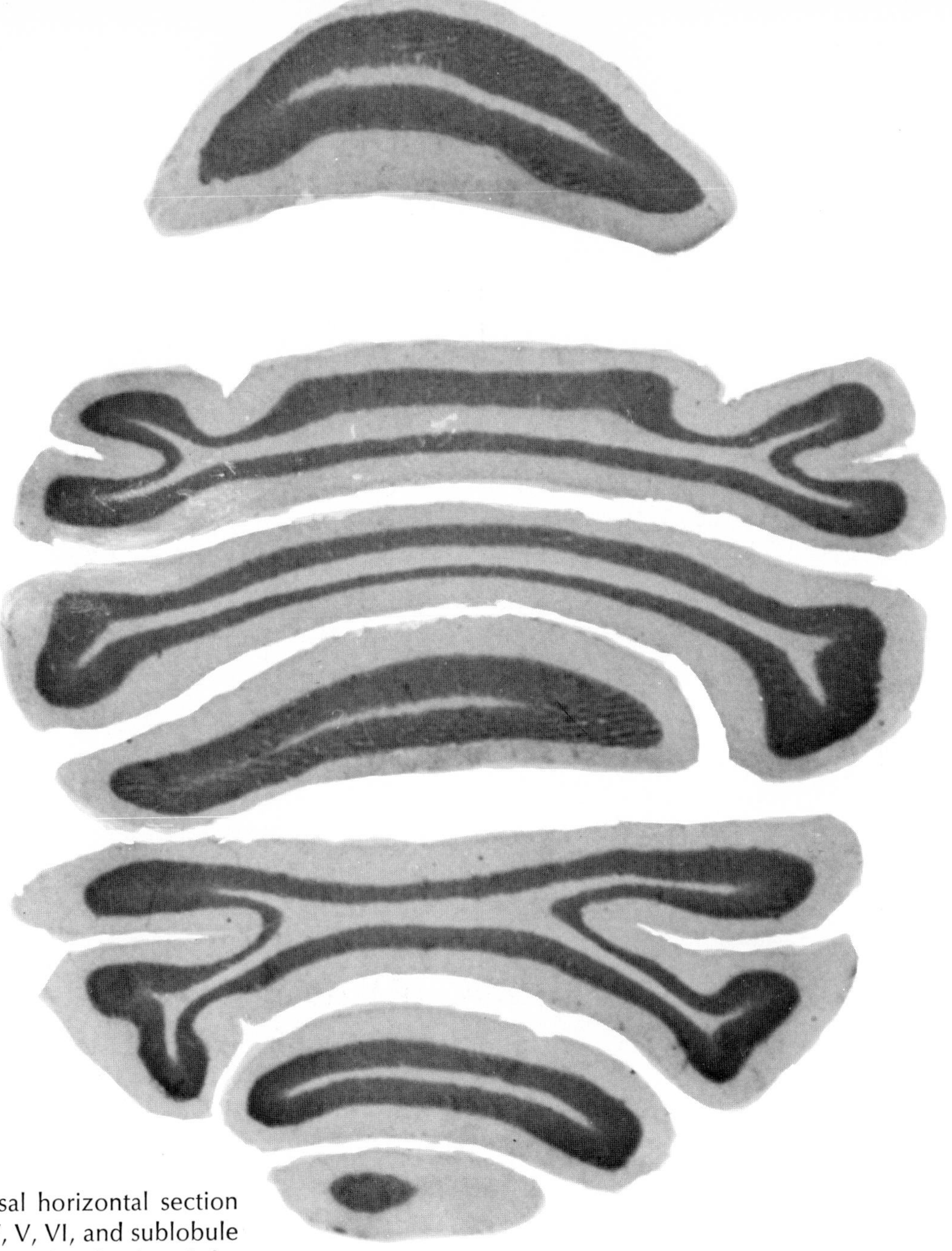

Figs. 43–44 This most dorsal horizontal section cuts through vermal lobules IV, V, VI, and sublobule VIIA. Folium V$_c$, which arises in the depths of the primary fissure, is shown reaching almost to the vermal surface. The planes of section of the horizontal series can be seen in Orientation Figures 11 and 12. *Nissl. X 12.*

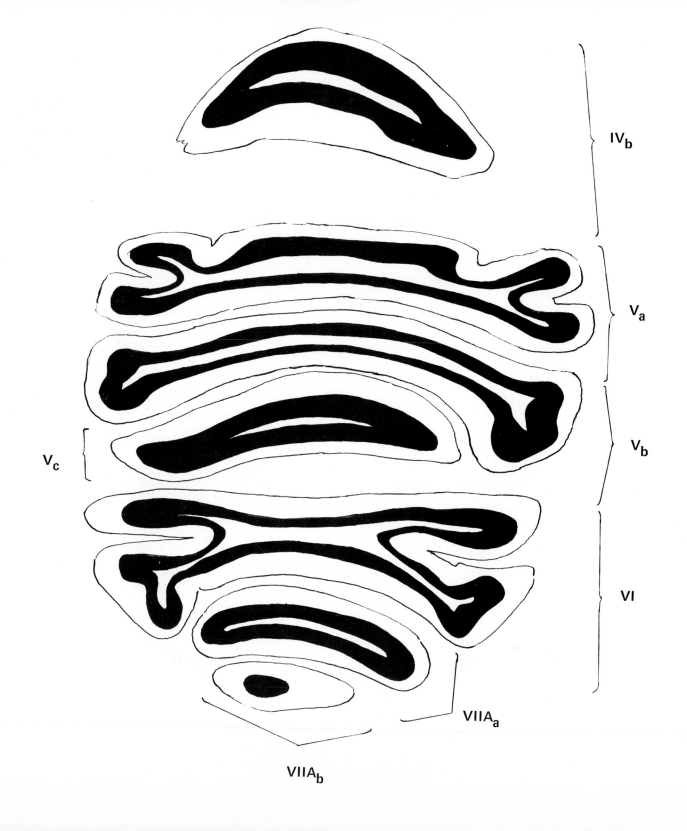

IV_b

V_a

V_b

V_c

VI

VIIA_a

VIIA_b

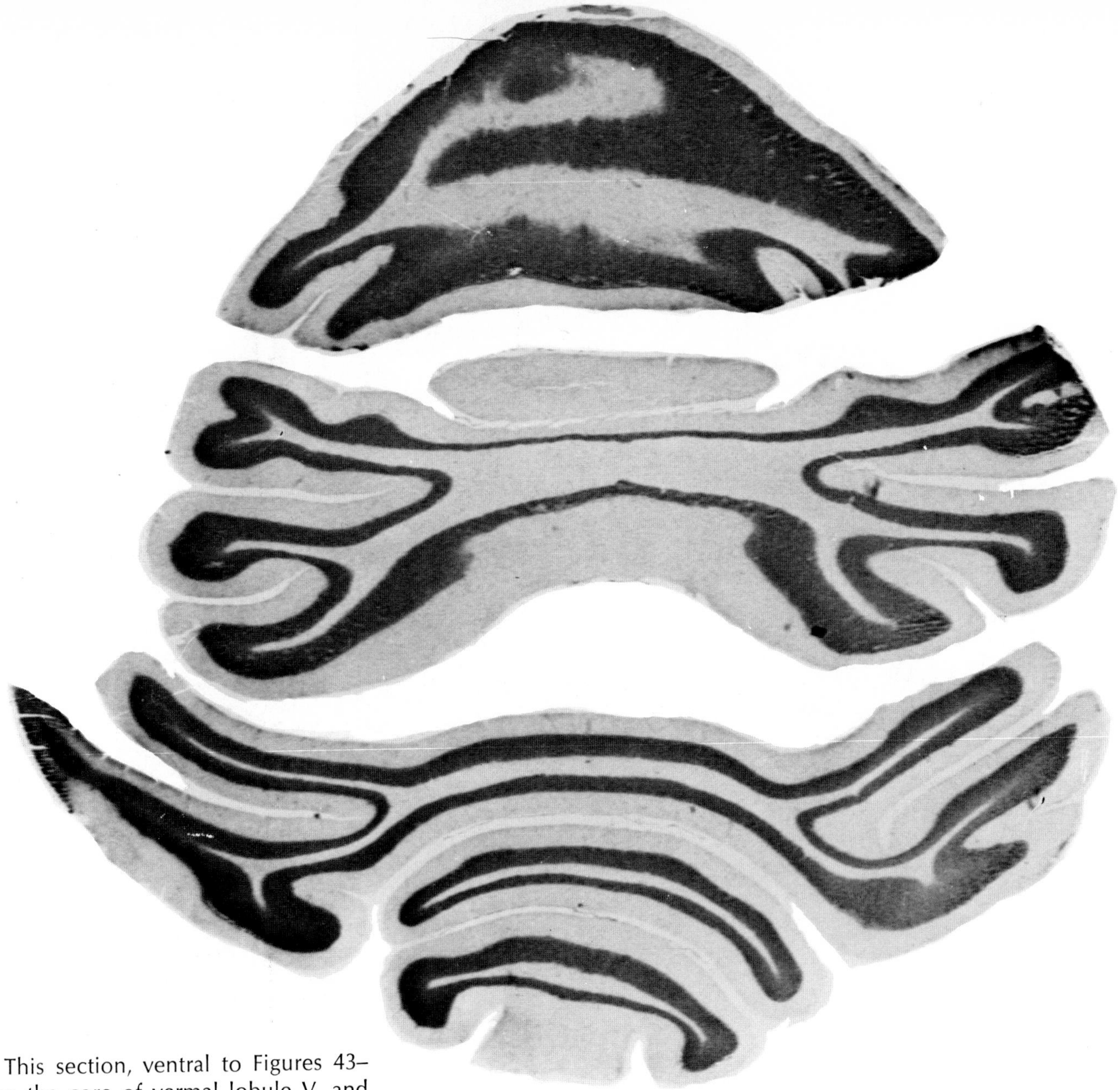

Figs. 45–46   This section, ventral to Figures 43–44, demonstrates the core of vermal lobule V, and its division into laminae V_a, V_b, and folium V_c. Lobules IV, VI, and sublobule VIIA are unchanged. The primary fissure is prominent between lobules V and VI.   Nissl. X 12.

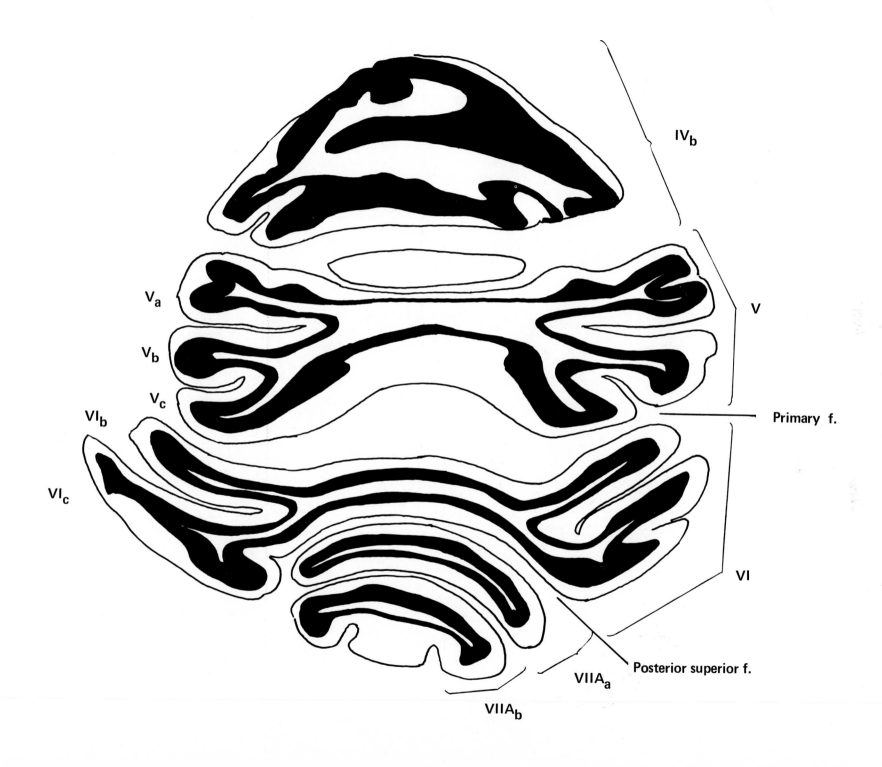

IV_b

V_a

V_b

V_c

VI_b

VI_c

V

Primary f.

VI

Posterior superior f.

VIIA_a

VIIA_b

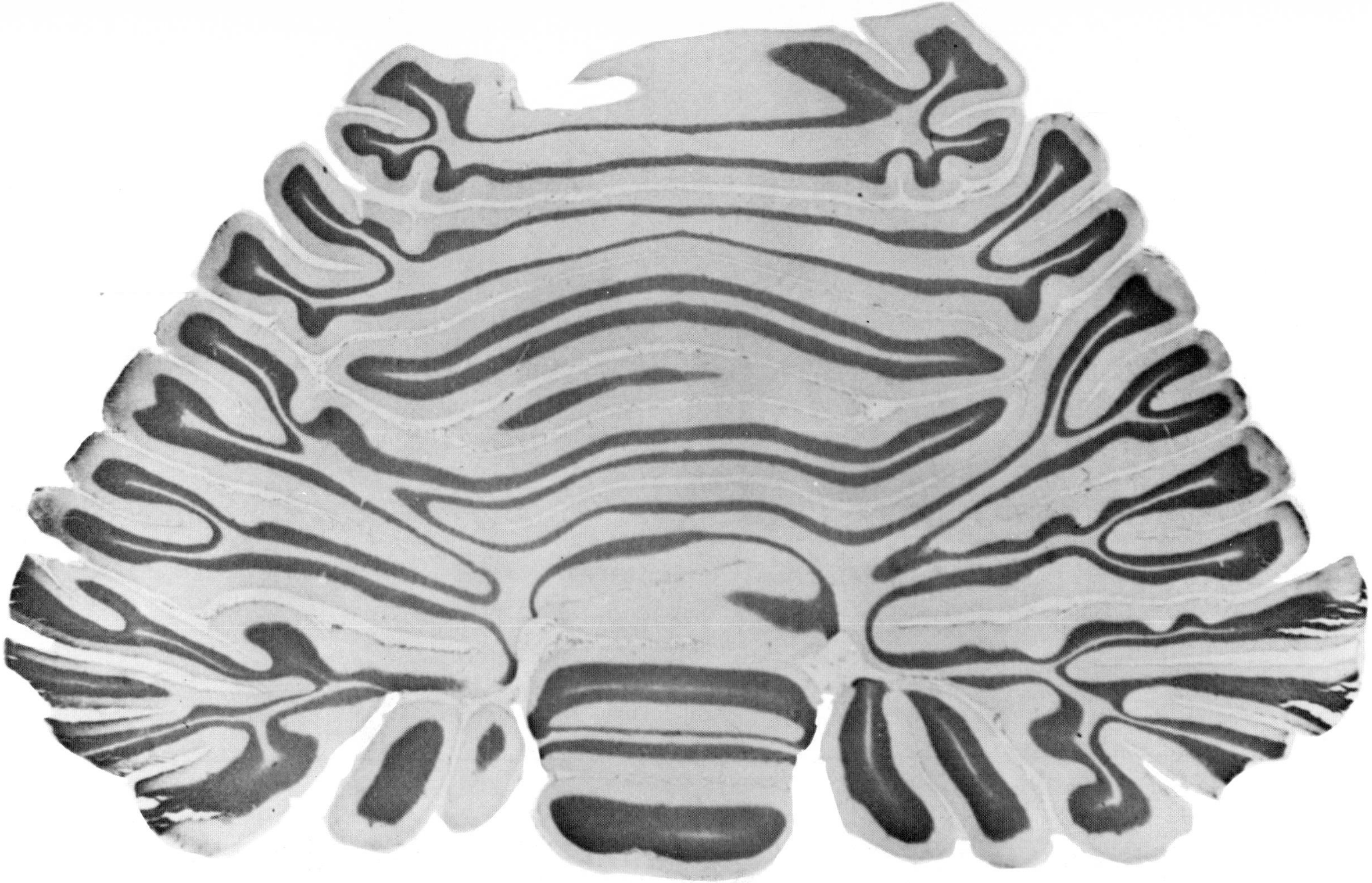

Figs. 47–48 This section through the upper third of the vermis reveals several important changes. The vermal core of lobule IV can be traced laterally to its two hemispheric laminae, IV$_a$ and IV$_b$. A similar configuration is noted for vermal lobule V and its laminae V$_a$ and V$_b$. Together the hemispheric folia of lobules IV and V constitute the anterior quadrangular lobule. Folia V$_d$, VI$_f$, and VI$_d$ can be seen adjacent to the primary fissure.

Vermal sublobule VIIA and lobule VI now have a single medullary core, which can be traced laterally into the hemispheres as the simple lobule whose four surface folia correspond to VI$_a$, VI$_{b-c}$, VIIA$_a$, and VIIA$_a$′. Sublobule VIIB, which, as noted in the Introduction, represents the most ventrocaudal folia of lobule VII, is shown. Vermal lobule VIIIA also is present at this level.

The ansiform lobule (**crus I** and **II**) occupies the most posterior regions of the section, and the continuity of its medullary core with that of lobule VII is demonstrated. The posterior superior fissure separates the simple lobule from the ansiform lobule in the hemispheres.   *Nissl. X 12.*

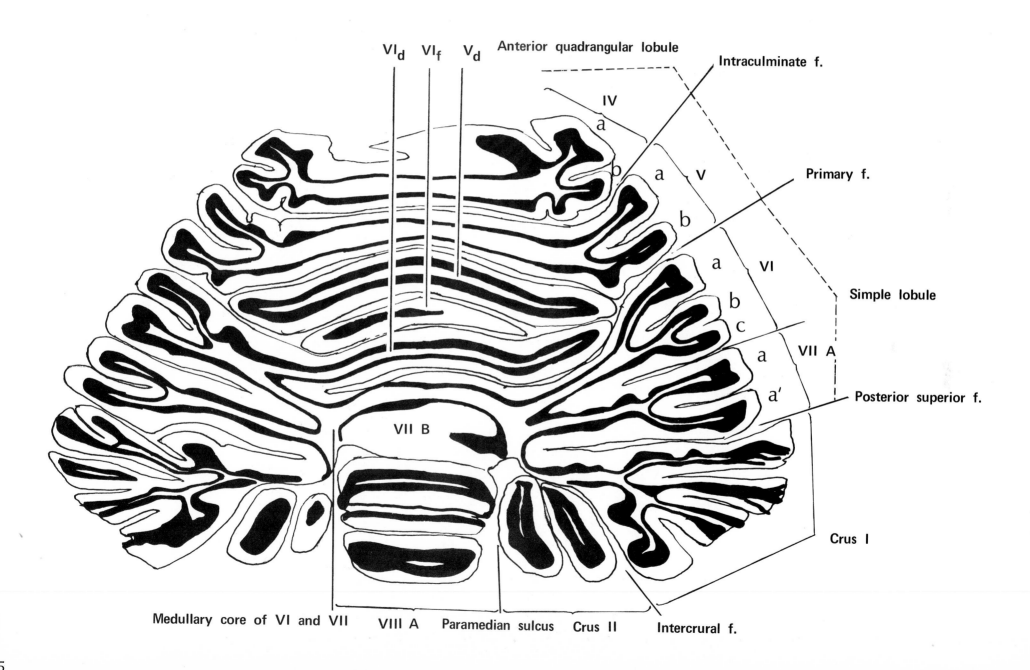

VI_d VI_f V_d

Anterior quadrangular lobule

Intraculminate f.

IV

a

b

a

V

b

Primary f.

a

VI

b

c

Simple lobule

a

VII A

a'

Posterior superior f.

VII B

Crus I

Medullary core of VI and VII   VIII A   Paramedian sulcus   Crus II   Intercrural f.

66

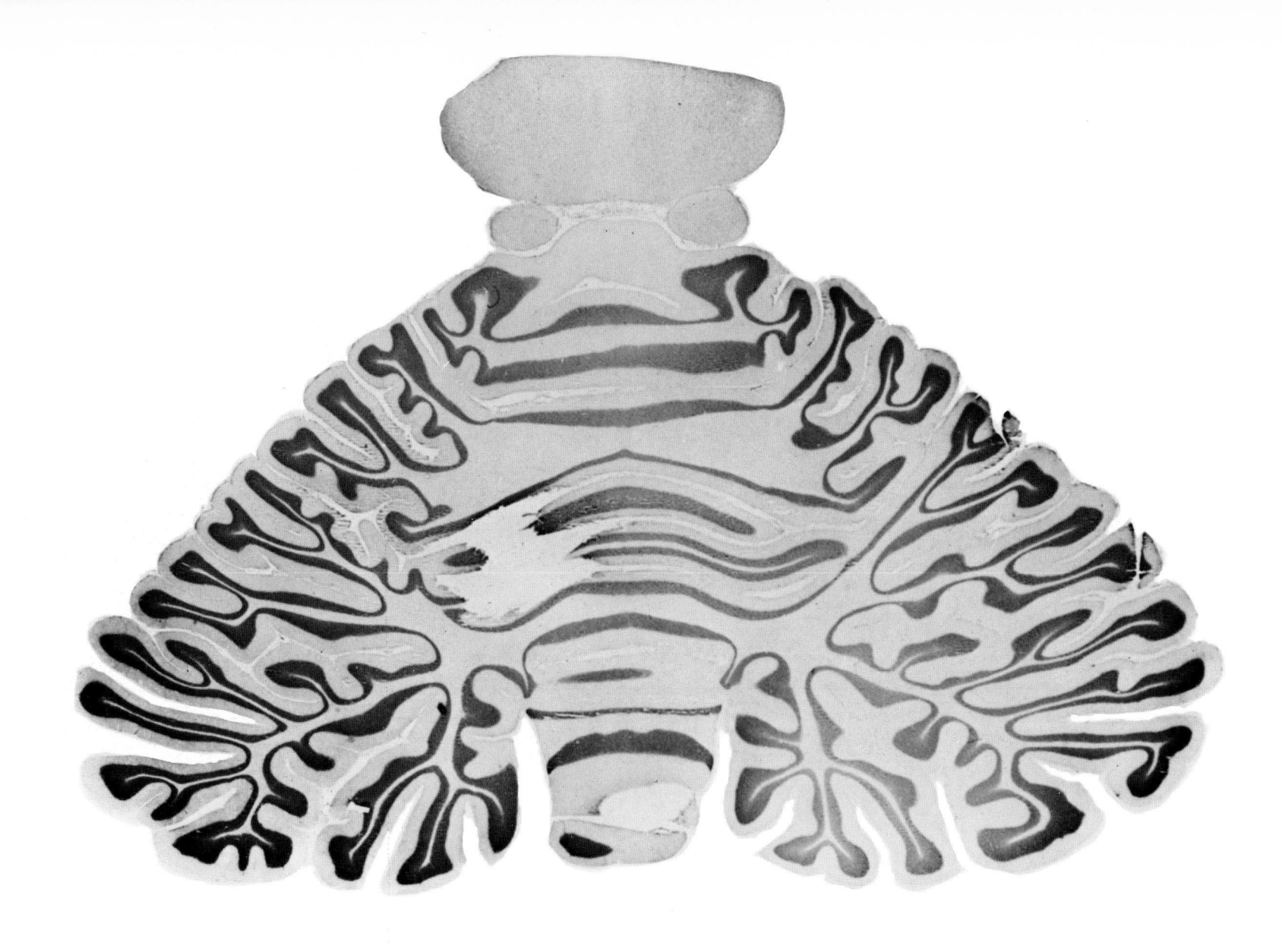

Figs. 49–50 This plane, ventral to Figures 47–48, reveals vermal lobule III and its hemispheric laminae III_a and III_b. A common medullary core for lobules IV and V is indicated, as it extends into its hemispheric counterpart, the anterior quadrangular lobule.

Folia V_e and VI_f lie in the primary fissure. The common medullary core for lobules VI and VII is again prominent, and this core can be seen extending anteriorly to form the simple lobule, and posteriorly to form the ansiform lobule. The division of the ansiform lobule into crus I and crus II on the basis of its two separate medullary cores is indicated. Vermal sublobule VIIIB also is present in this plane. *Nissl. X 6.*

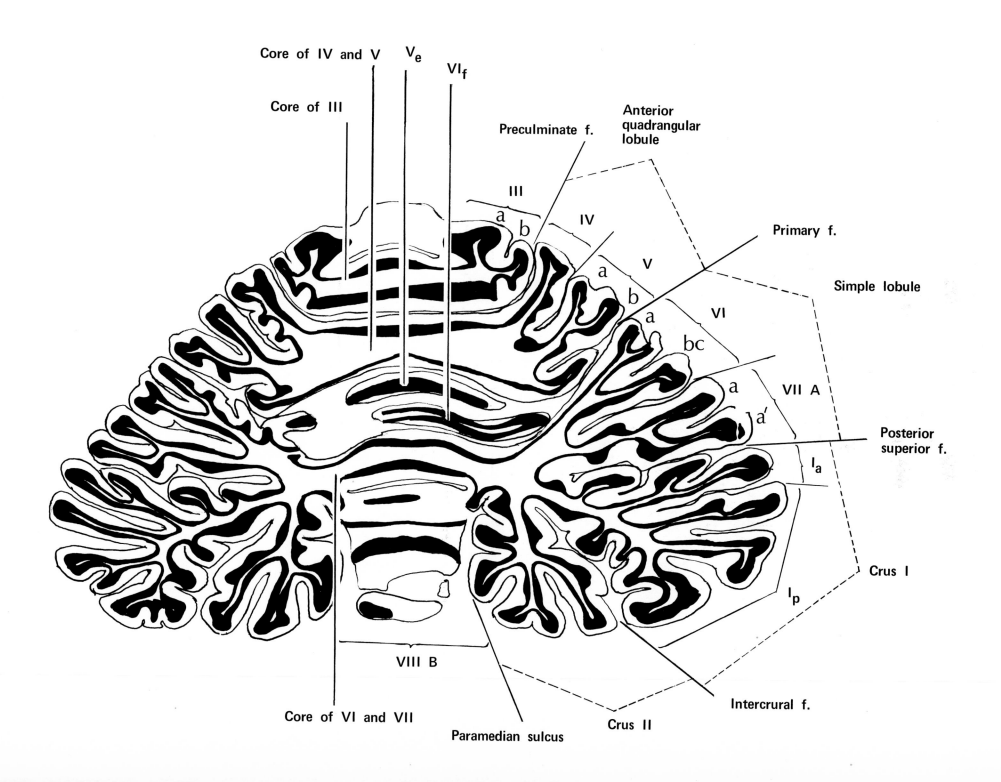

Core of IV and V   V$_e$ VI$_f$

Core of III

Anterior quadrangular lobule

Preculminate f.

III

a b   IV

V
a
b
a   VI
bc

Primary f.

Simple lobule

VII A
a
a′

Posterior superior f.

I$_a$

Crus I

I$_p$

Intercrural f.

VIII B

Core of VI and VII

Paramedian sulcus

Crus II

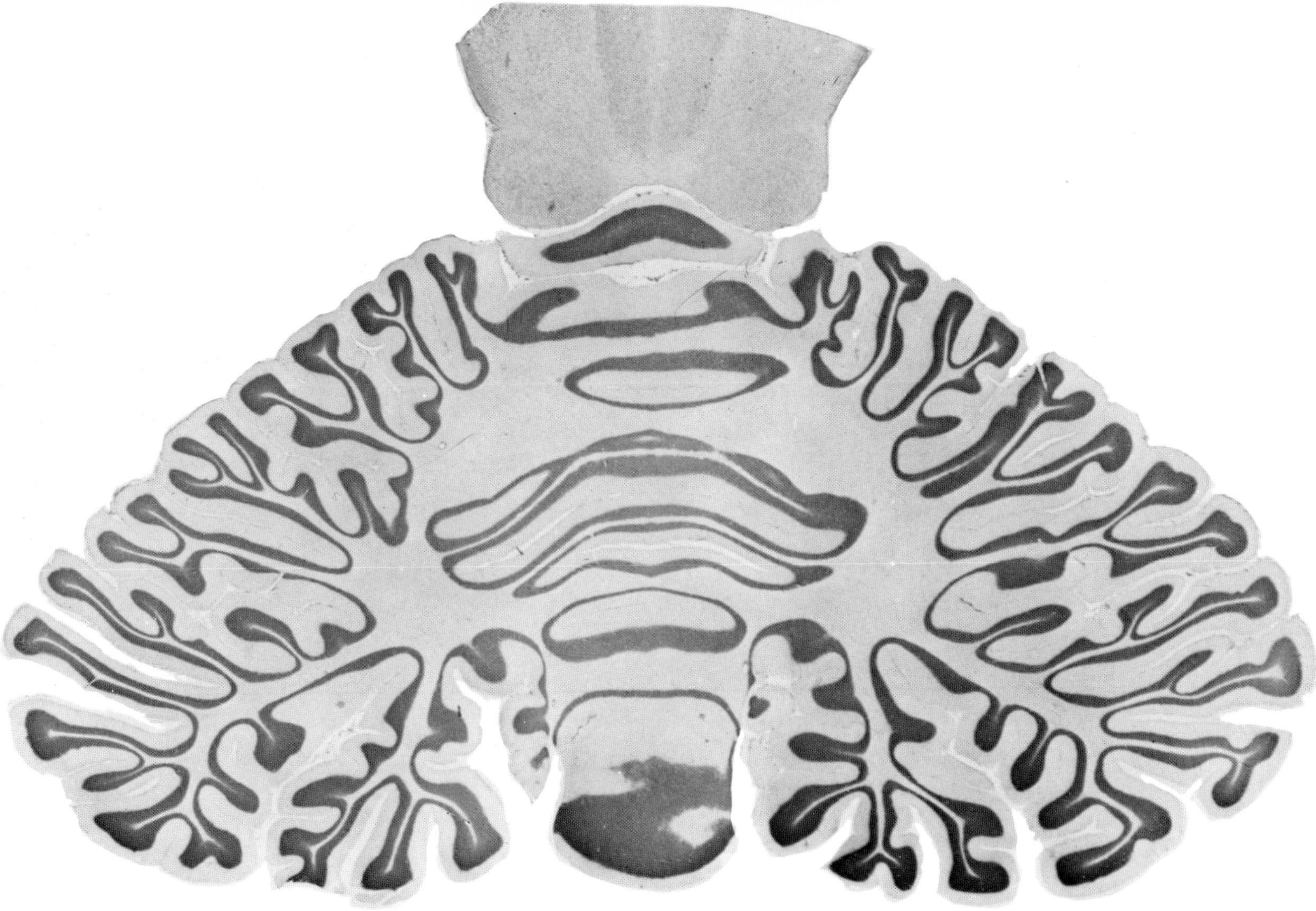

Figs. 51–52 In this section vermal lamina II$_b$ is first noted. Vermal lobules III, IV, and V can be seen merging into a single medullary core. The relationship of folium V$_e$ to the core of lobule V, and of folium VI$_f$ to the core of lobule VI in the depths of the primary fissure is indicated.

Only the medullary core of vermal lobule VIII can be seen. The first traces of the paramedian lobule appear lateral to the core of vermal lobule VIII in the depths of the paramedian sulcus. The most dorsal folia of vermal IX$_a$ appear caudal to the medullary core of vermal lobule VIII.

The most anterior folia of crus I constitute crus I$_a$, while the bulk of crus I lies posteriorly (**crus I$_p$**). *Nissl. X 6.*

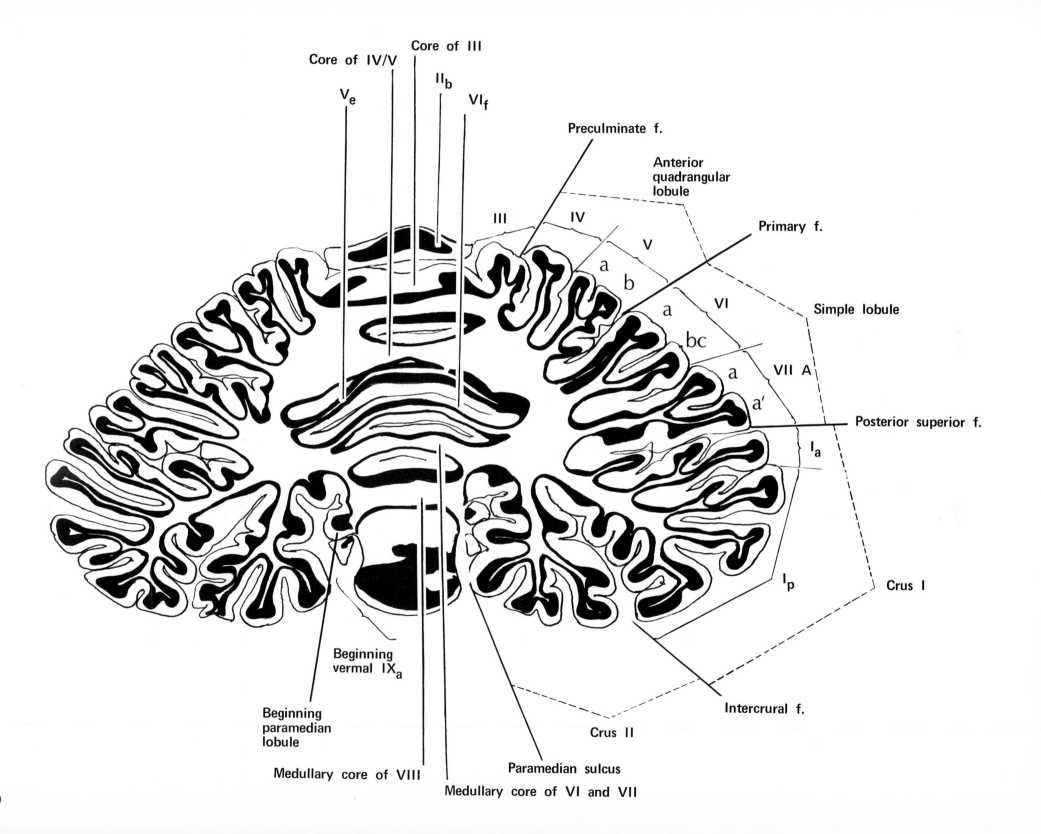

Core of IV/V

Core of III

V_e

II_b

VI_f

Preculminate f.

Anterior quadrangular lobule

III

IV

V

a

b

a

bc

a

a'

Primary f.

Simple lobule

VI

VII A

Posterior superior f.

I_a

I_p

Crus I

Intercrural f.

Crus II

Paramedian sulcus

Medullary core of VI and VII

Medullary core of VIII

Beginning vermal IX_a

Beginning paramedian lobule

69

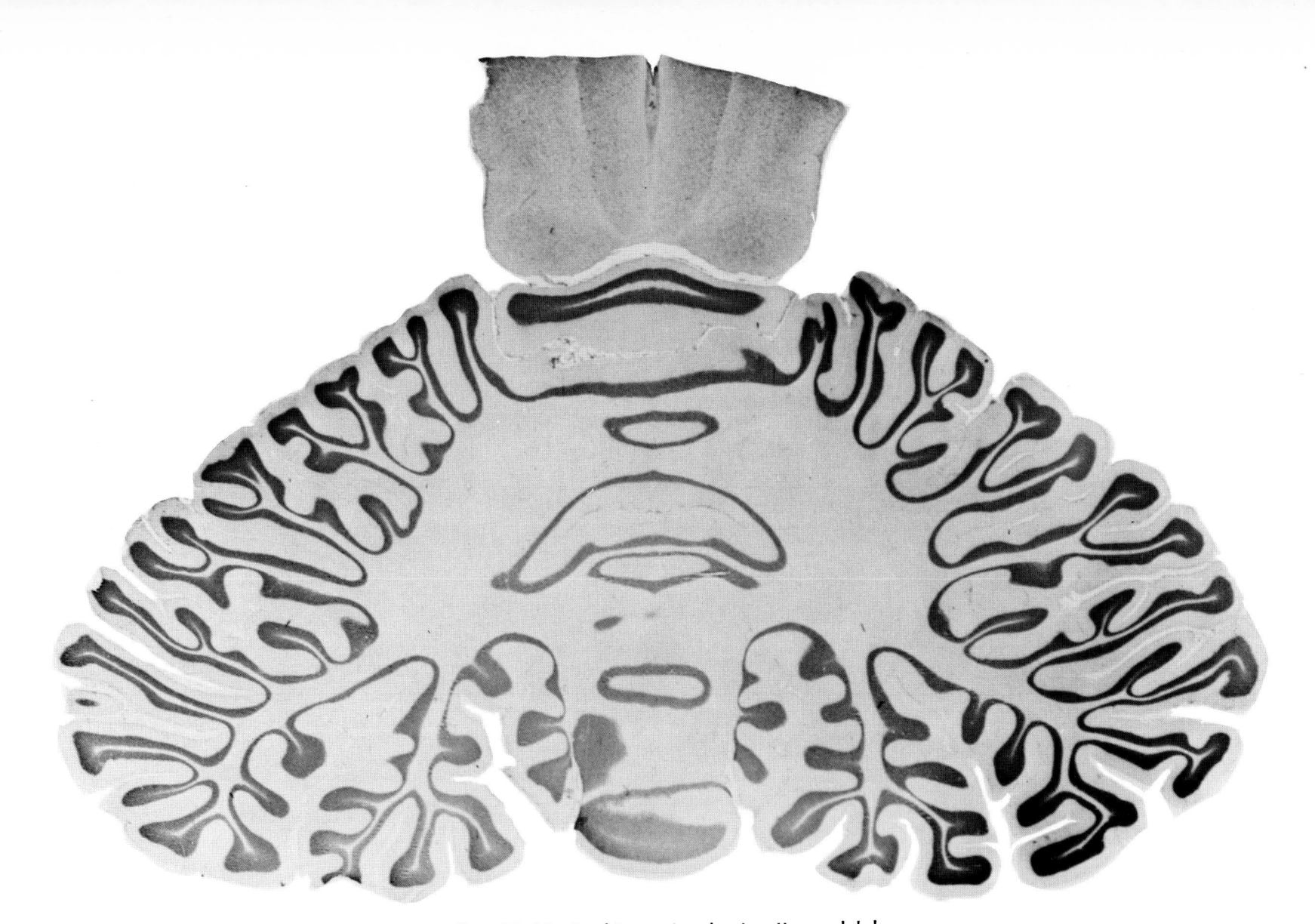

Figs. 53–54 In this section lamina II$_b$, and lobules III, IV, and V are unchanged. The medullary cores of vermal lobules VI, VII, and VIII have merged, while the paramedian lobule and its continuity with vermal lobule VIII has become more prominent. The simple lobule and ansiform lobule occupy most of the lateral extent of the hemispheres, and folium VI$_f$ can be seen in the most ventral part of the primary fissure. Vermal lamina IX$_a$ lies in the posterior vermis at this level. *Nissl.* X 6.

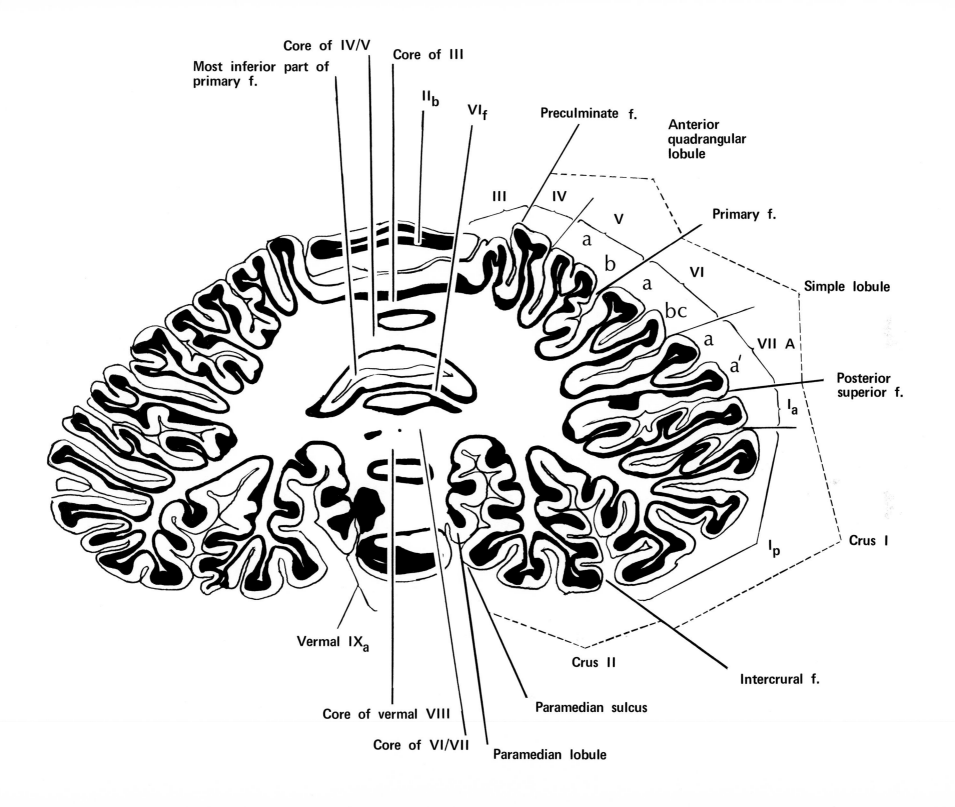

Most inferior part of primary f.

Core of IV/V

Core of III

II_b

VI_f

Preculminate f.

Anterior quadrangular lobule

III

IV

V

a

b

a

bc

a

a'

Primary f.

VI

VII A

Simple lobule

Posterior superior f.

I_a

I_p

Crus I

Vermal IX_a

Crus II

Intercrural f.

Core of vermal VIII

Core of VI/VII

Paramedian sulcus

Paramedian lobule

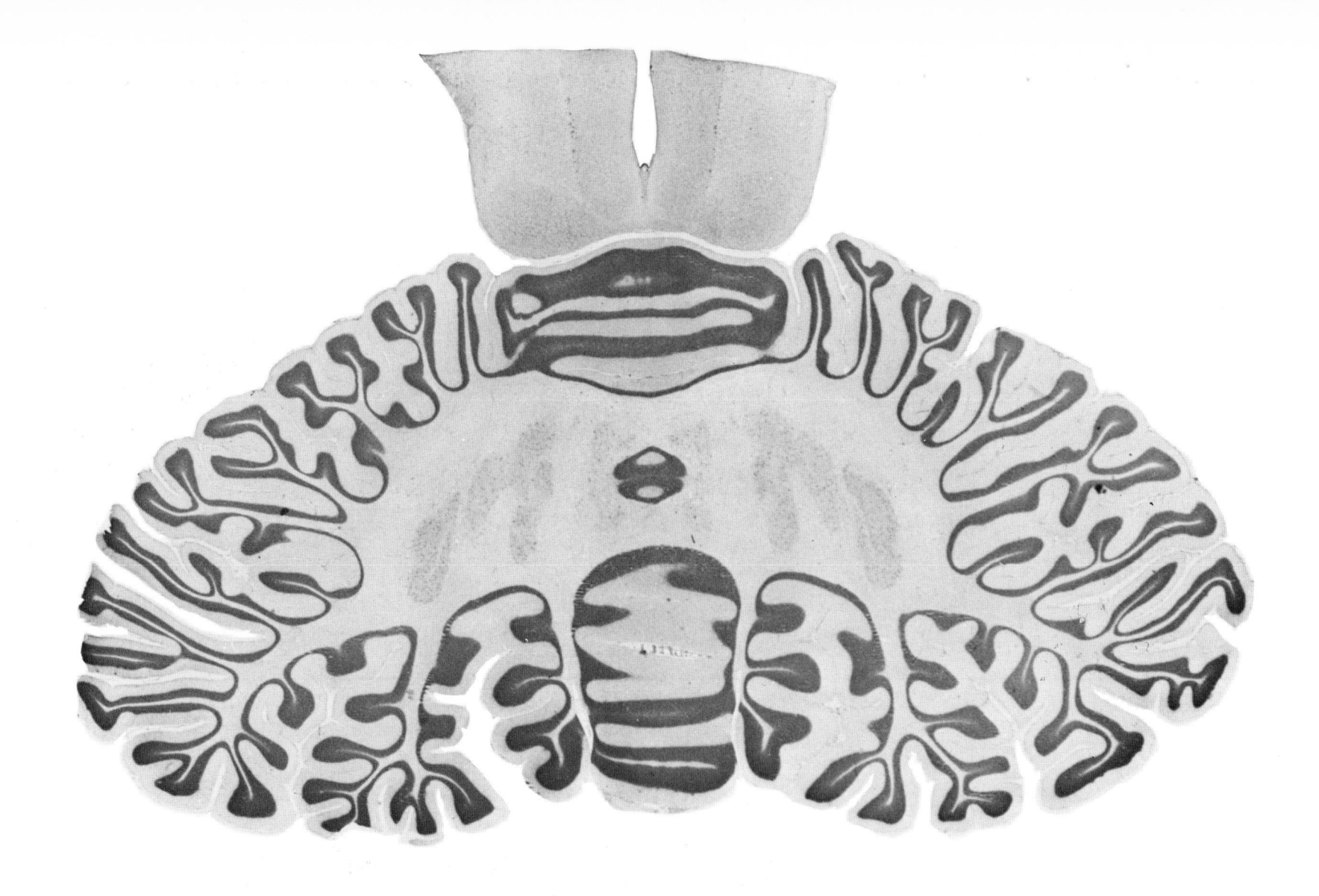

Figs. 55–56 The last trace of the primary fissure appears in this section. Lamina II$_b$ is prominent and only the medullary core of vermal lobules III, IV, and V can be seen. The central (**III**) and anterior quadrangular lobules (**IV** and **V**) occupy the hemispheres anteriorly, but are becoming overshadowed by the large lateral extent of the simple and ansiform lobules.

The paramedian lobule and its continuity with the medullary core of vermal lobule VIII is again noted. The dentate (**DN**), posterior interposed (**PIN**), anterior interposed (**AIN**), and fastigial nuclei (**FN**) are indicated in the central medullary substance. *Nissl. X 6.*

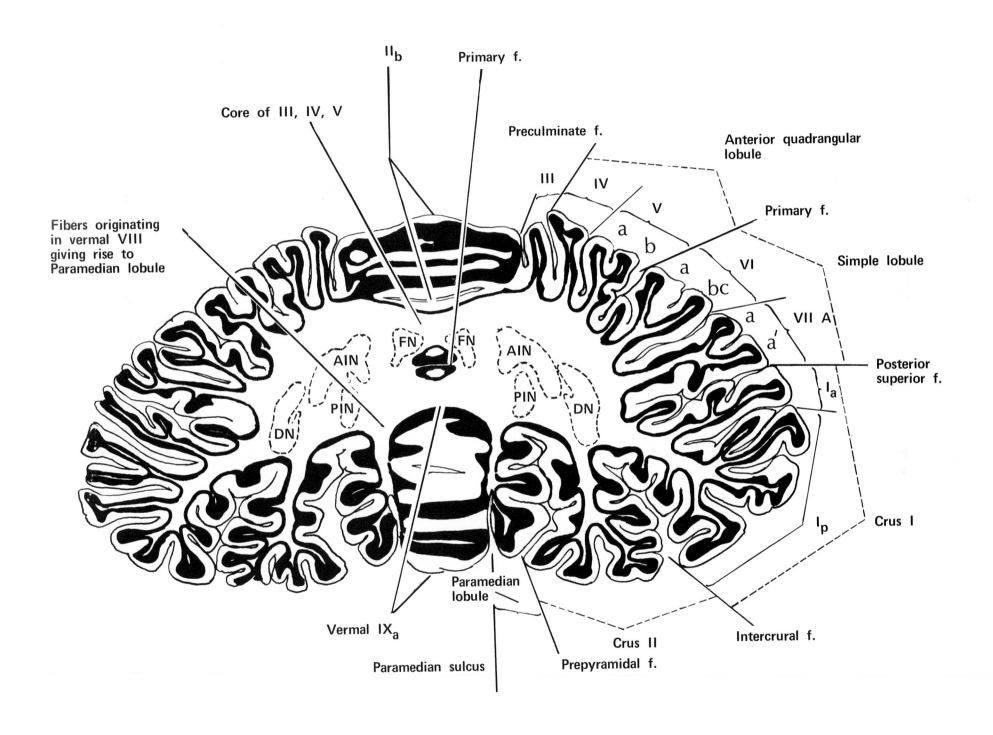

II_b

Primary f.

Core of III, IV, V

Preculminate f.

Anterior quadrangular
lobule

III   IV

V

a

b

Primary f.

a

VI

Simple lobule

bc

a

Fibers originating
in vermal VIII
giving rise to
Paramedian lobule

VII A

a'

FN   FN

AIN

AIN

Posterior
superior f.

PIN

PIN   DN

I_a

DN

I_p

Crus I

Vermal IX_a

Paramedian
lobule

Crus II

Intercrural f.

Paramedian sulcus

Prepyramidal f.

73

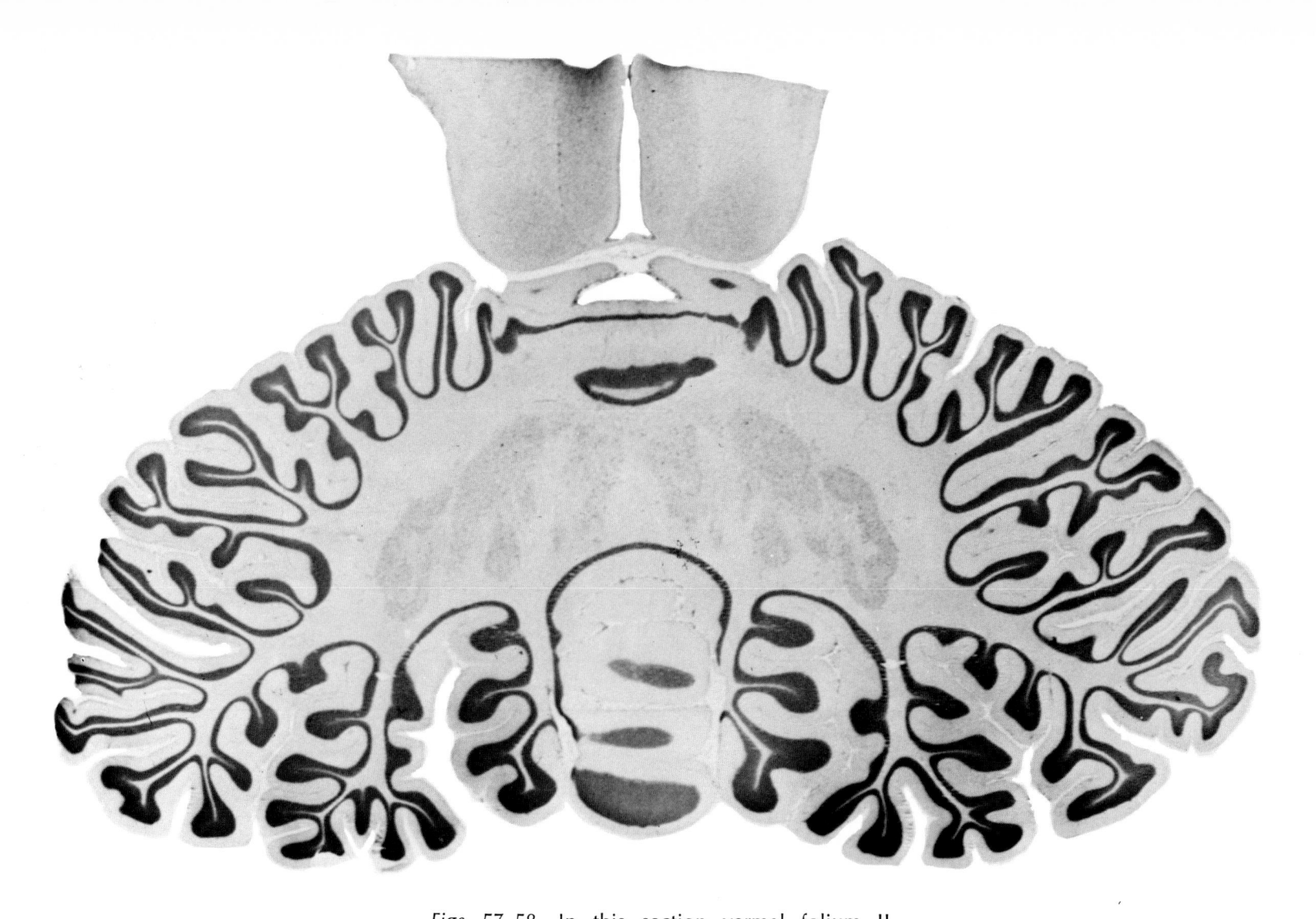

Figs. 57–58 In this section vermal folium II$_a$ appears and lamina II$_b$ is no longer present in the vermis, but its hemispheric counterpart can be seen laterally. This lateral extension of lamina II$_b$ contributes to the central lobule along with a folium from vermal lobule III. The anterior quadrangular lobule is unchanged, as are the simple and ansiform lobules. The two divisions of crus II (**II$_a$** and **II$_p$**) are shown, and the four deep cerebellar nuclei are indicated.   *Nissl.* X 6.

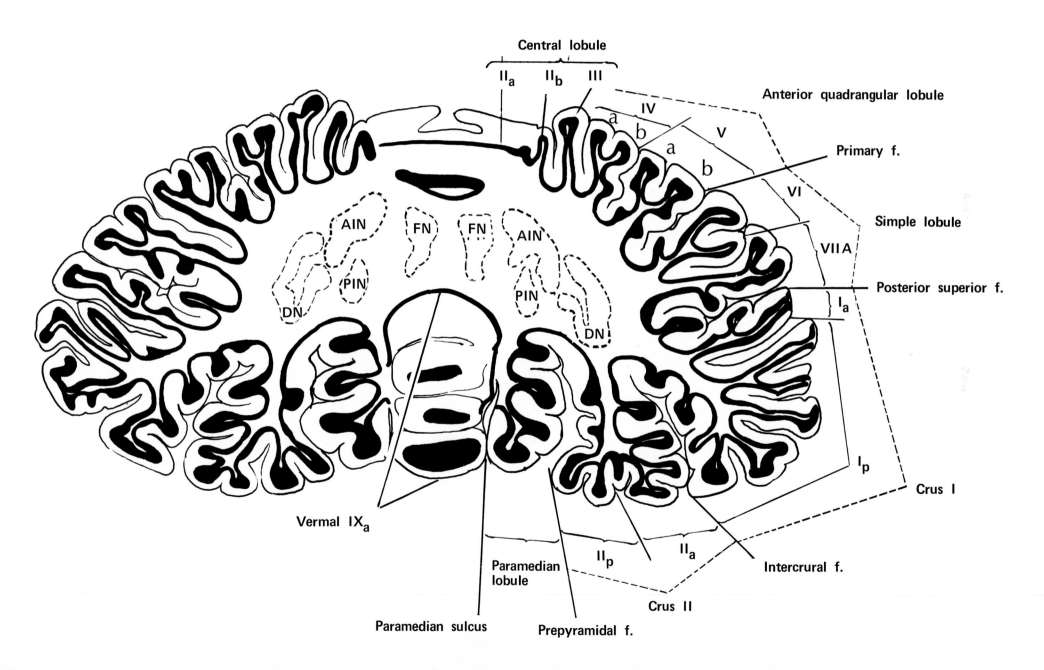

Central lobule

II_a II_b III

Anterior quadrangular lobule

IV
a
b
b
a
V

Primary f.

VI

Simple lobule

AIN   FN   FN   AIN

VIIA

PIN   PIN

Posterior superior f.

DN   DN

I_a

I_p

Crus I

Vermal IX_a

II_p   II_a

Intercrural f.

Paramedian
lobule

Crus II

Paramedian sulcus   Prepyramidal f.

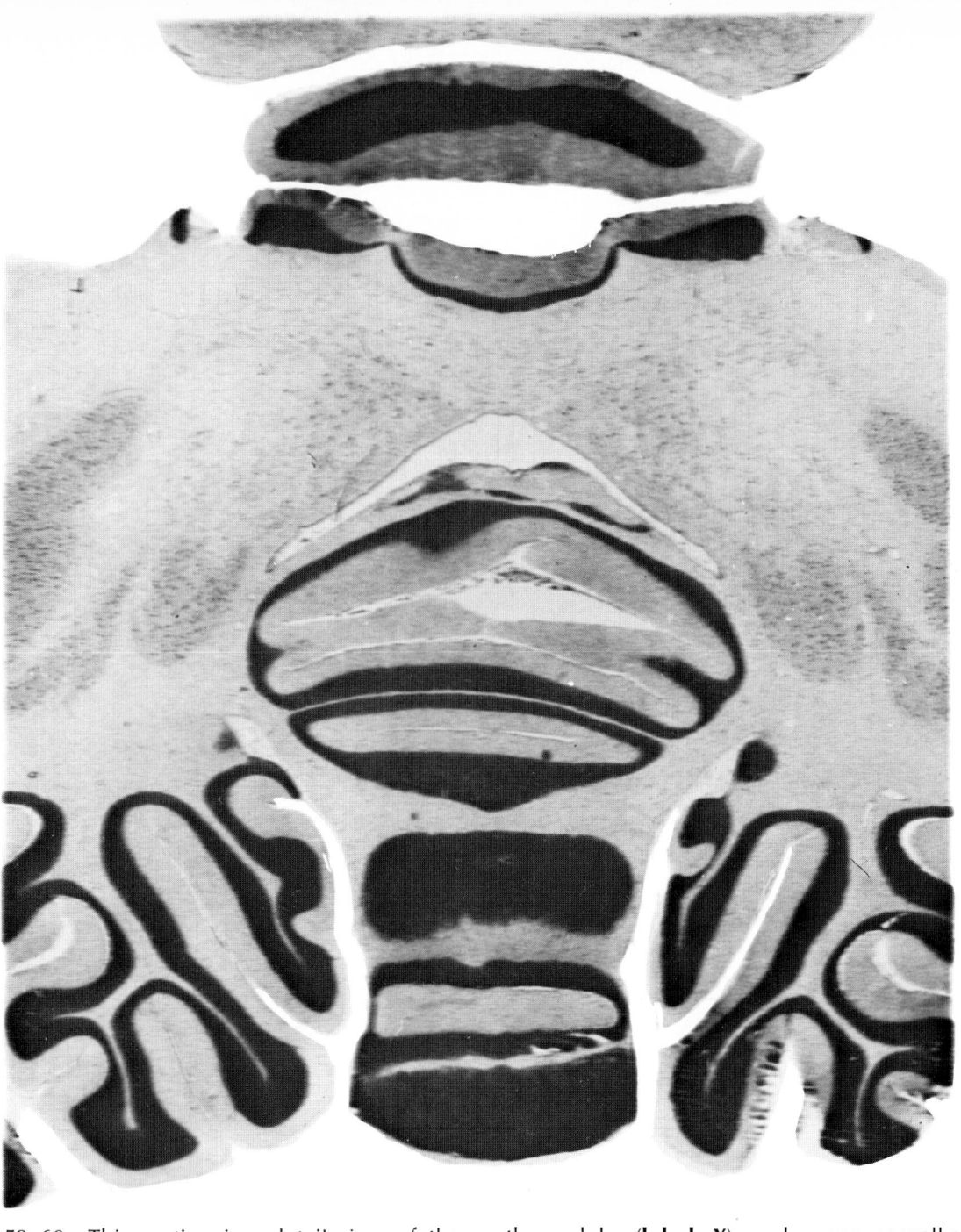

Figs. 59–60 This section is a detail view of the central medullary substance of the cerebellum through the roof of the fourth ventricle. The inferior portion of folium II_a, and the core of lamina I_{b-c} are present anteriorly. The approximate positions of the fastigial (**FN**), dentate (**DN**), and posterior interposed (**PIN**) nuclei are noted. The medullary core of the nodulus (**lobule X**) can be seen, as well as lobule IX, with its laminae $IX_{b,c,d}$ merging with lamina IX_a.

In this plane fibers from the medullary core of vermal IX spread laterally and these fibers ultimately give rise to the peduncle of the paraflocculus. The lobules of the hemisphere undergo little change in this section and in those adjacent to it.   *Nissl. X 12.*

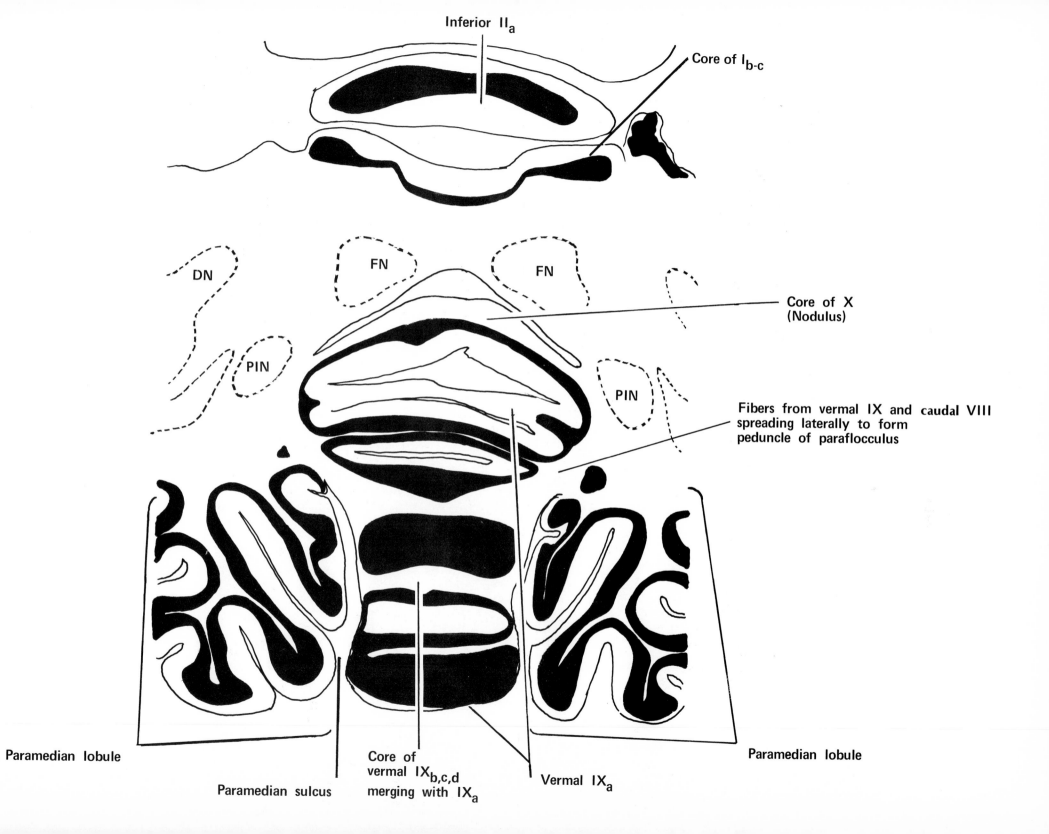

Inferior II_a

Core of I_{b-c}

DN

FN

FN

Core of X
(Nodulus)

PIN

PIN

Fibers from vermal IX and caudal VIII
spreading laterally to form
peduncle of paraflocculus

Paramedian lobule

Paramedian lobule

Core of
vermal IX$_{b,c,d}$
merging with IX$_a$

Paramedian sulcus

Vermal IX$_a$

Figs. 61–62 This is another detail view of a cerebellar section slightly ventral to Figures 59–60. The core of lamina I$_{b-c}$ and the core of folium I$_a$ are noted, as are the folia of the nodulus. Fibers originating from the medullary core of the nodulus (**lobule X**) can be seen spreading laterally, where they ultimately form the peduncle of the flocculus. Vermal IX and its subdivisions are prominent, as in the previous section. The fastigial (**FN**), posterior interposed (**PIN**), and dentate (**DN**) nuclei are indicated. *Nissl. X 8.*

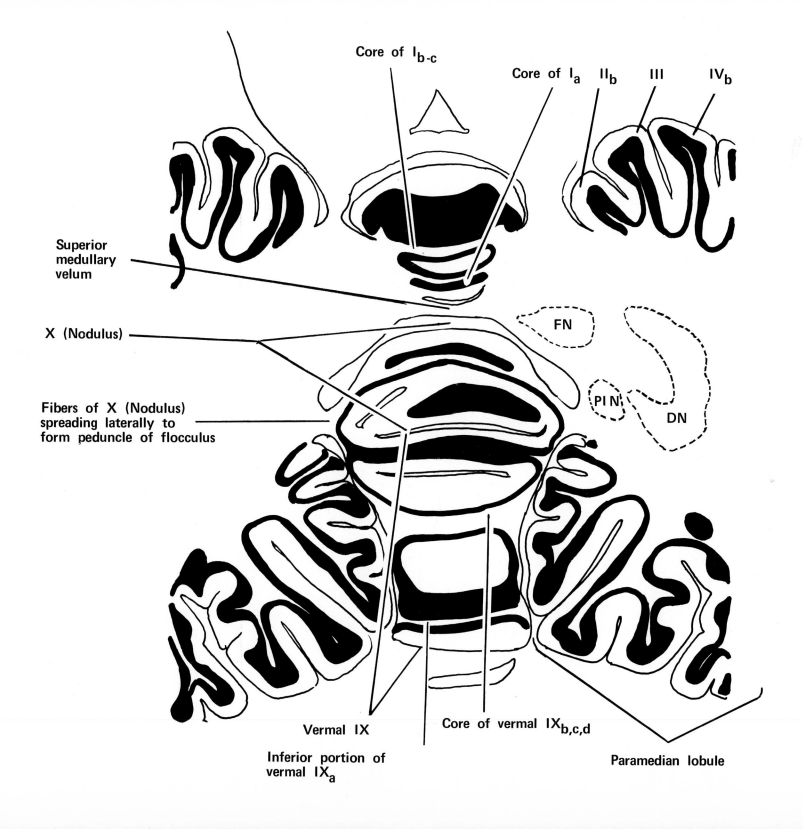

Core of I$_{b-c}$

Core of I$_a$ II$_b$ III   IV$_b$

Superior
medullary
velum

X (Nodulus)

Fibers of X (Nodulus)
spreading laterally to
form peduncle of flocculus

FN

PI N

DN

Vermal IX

Core of vermal IX$_{b,c,d}$

Inferior portion of
vermal IX$_a$

Paramedian lobule

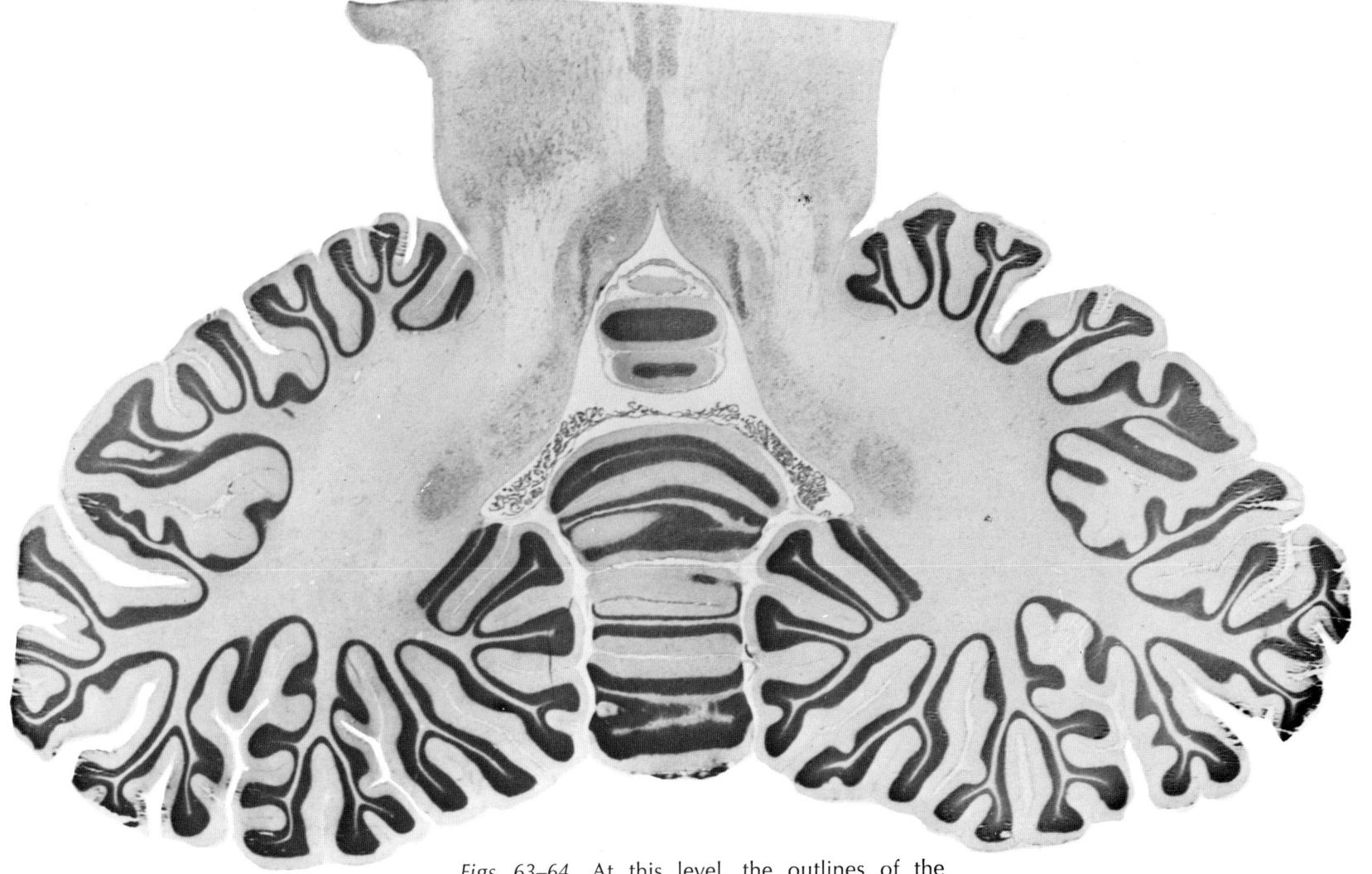

Figs. 63–64 At this level, the outlines of the fourth ventricle and its choroid plexus are visible, and the vermal lobules I (**lingula**) and X (**nodulus**) can be seen protruding into the fourth ventricle. Inferior portions of vermal IX are present, and the paramedian lobule has become more prominent.

Only the anterior quadrangular lobule remains in the anterior cerebellar hemisphere. The simple lobule and ansiform lobule are unchanged, although in crus II the division between II$_p$ and II$_a$ is more distinct. Only the dentate nucleus (**DN**) is present at this level in the central medullary substance. *Nissl. X 6.*

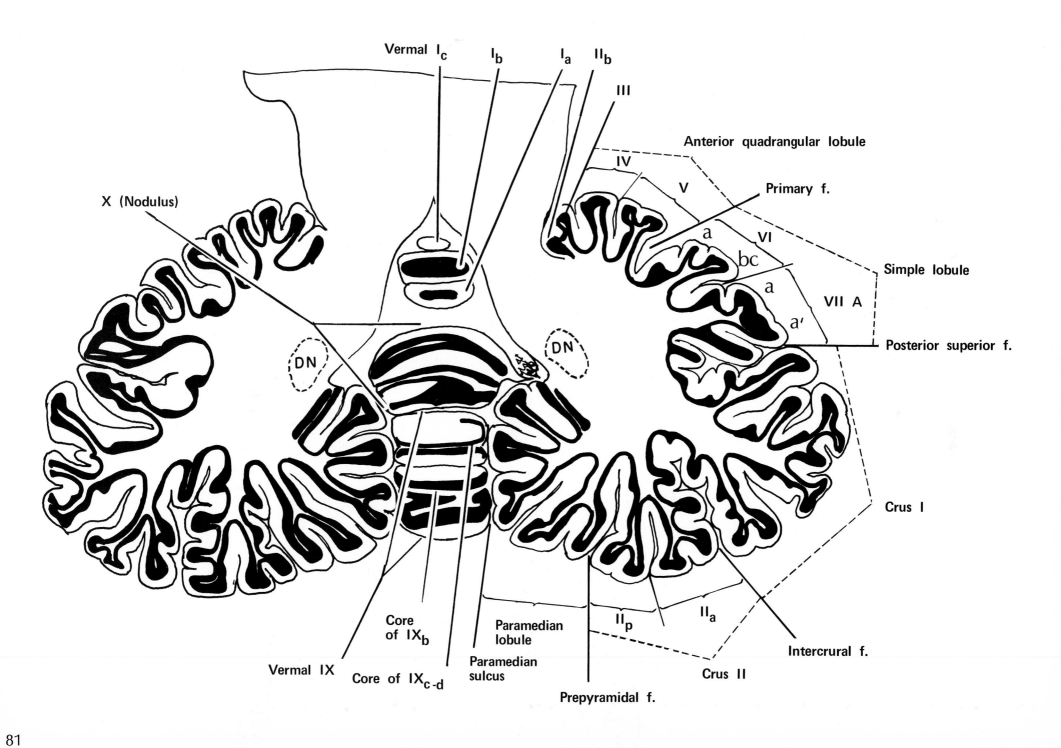

Vermal I$_c$
I$_b$
I$_a$
II$_b$
III
Anterior quadrangular lobule
IV
V
Primary f.
a
VI
bc
Simple lobule
a
VII A
a'
Posterior superior f.
X (Nodulus)
DN
DN
Crus I
Core of IX$_b$
Paramedian lobule
II$_p$
II$_a$
Intercrural f.
Vermal IX
Core of IX$_{c-d}$
Paramedian sulcus
Crus II
Prepyramidal f.

81

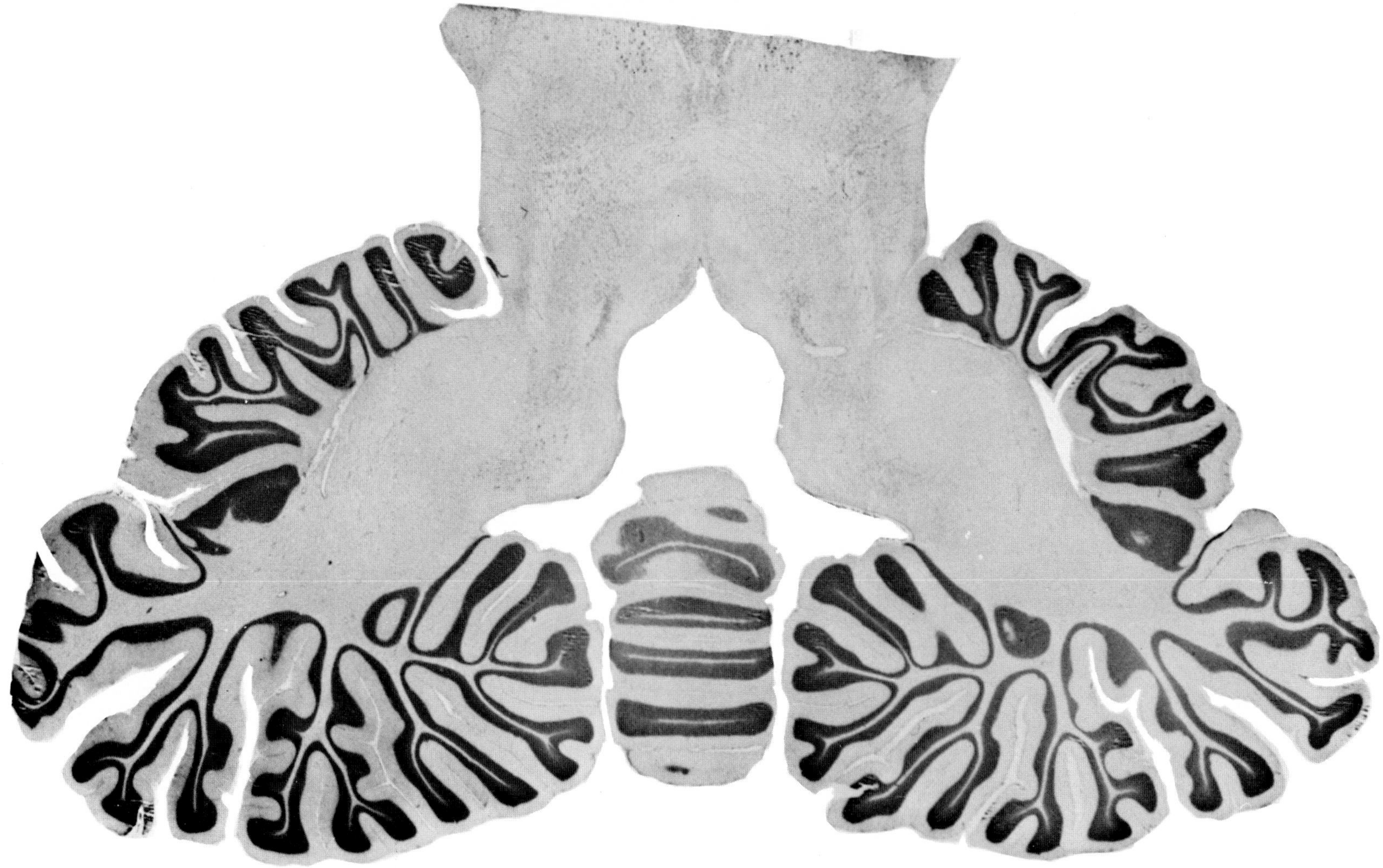

Figs. 65–66 At this level both the anterior quadrangular and simple lobules are disappearing from
view. Crus I$_a$ has disappeared, but the paramedian
lobule and the remainder of the ansiform lobule are
still prominent. The inferior folia of vermal lobule
IX are identified, as are the folia of the nodulus. The
superior cerebellar peduncles can be seen coursing
from each hemispheric core into the rostral brain
stem. *Nissl. X 6.*

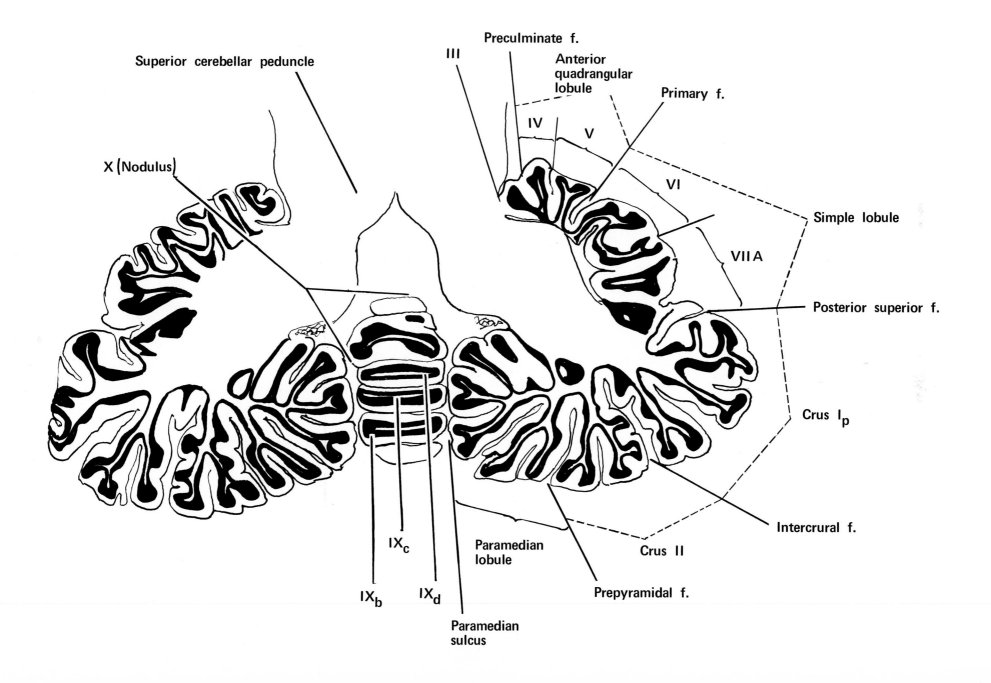

Superior cerebellar peduncle

Preculminate f.

III

Anterior quadrangular lobule

Primary f.

IV

V

VI

X (Nodulus)

Simple lobule

VII A

Posterior superior f.

Crus I$_p$

Intercrural f.

IX$_c$

Paramedian lobule

Crus II

IX$_b$

IX$_d$

Prepyramidal f.

Paramedian sulcus

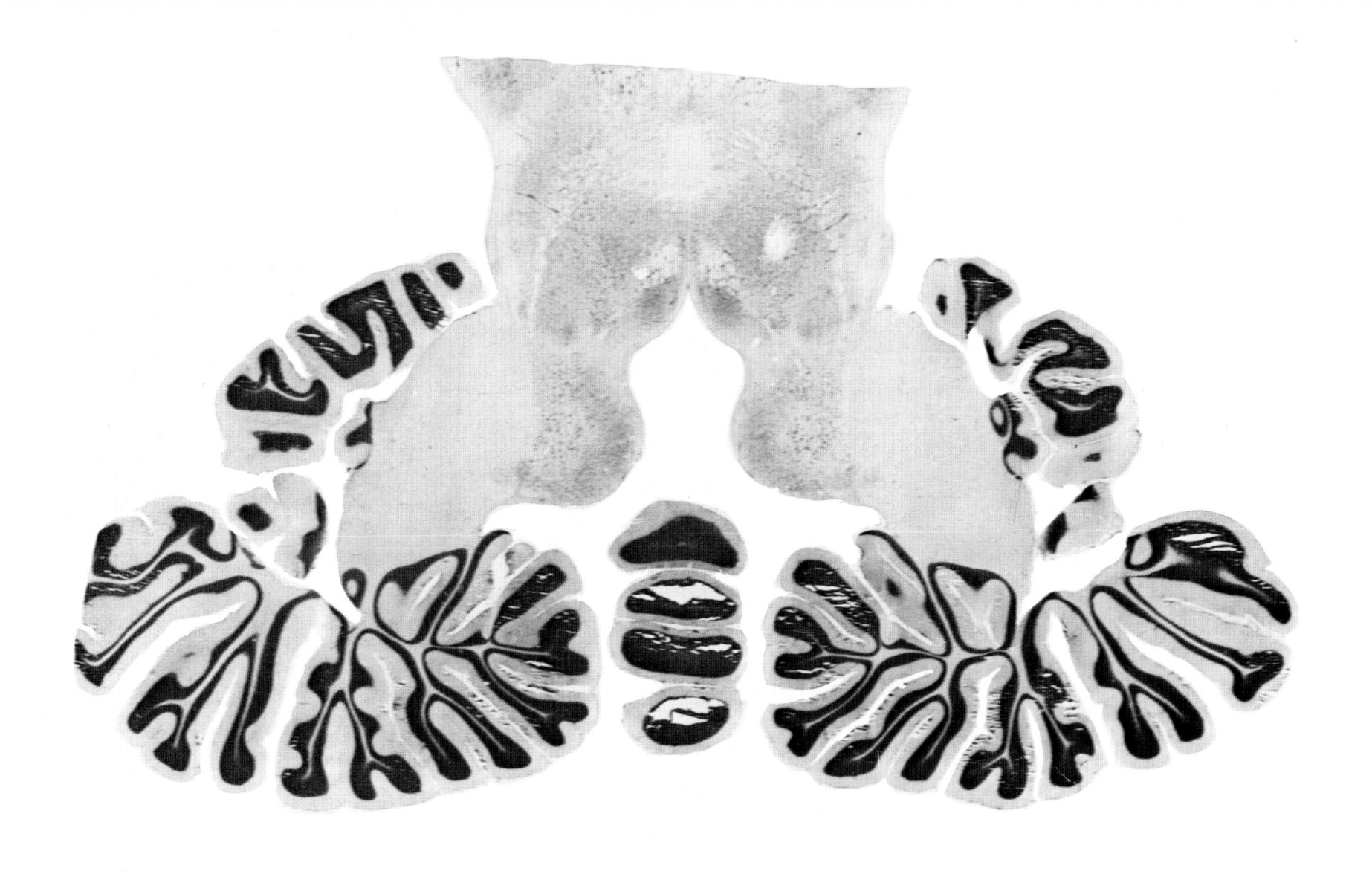

Figs. 67–68 At this level the first traces of the dorsal paraflocculus come into view. The most ventral folia of the nodulus and uvula are indicated. Crus I$_p$, crus II, and the paramedian lobule occupy the posterolateral aspect of the hemispheres. *Nissl. X 6.*

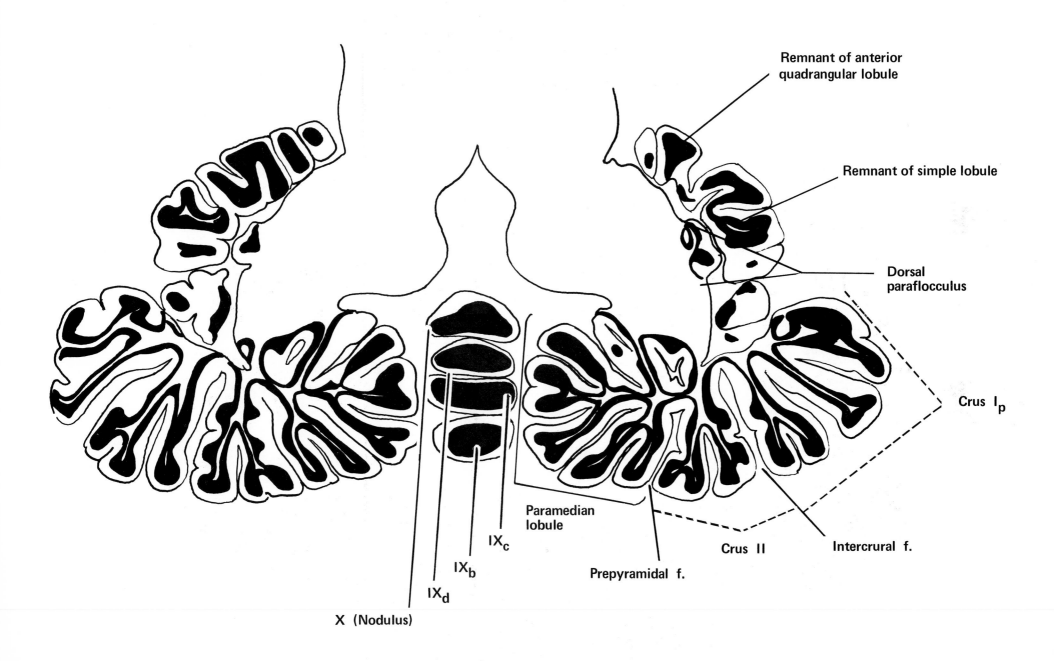

Remnant of anterior quadrangular lobule

Remnant of simple lobule

Dorsal paraflocculus

Crus I$_p$

Intercrural f.

Crus II

Prepyramidal f.

Paramedian lobule

IX$_c$

IX$_b$

IX$_d$

X (Nodulus)

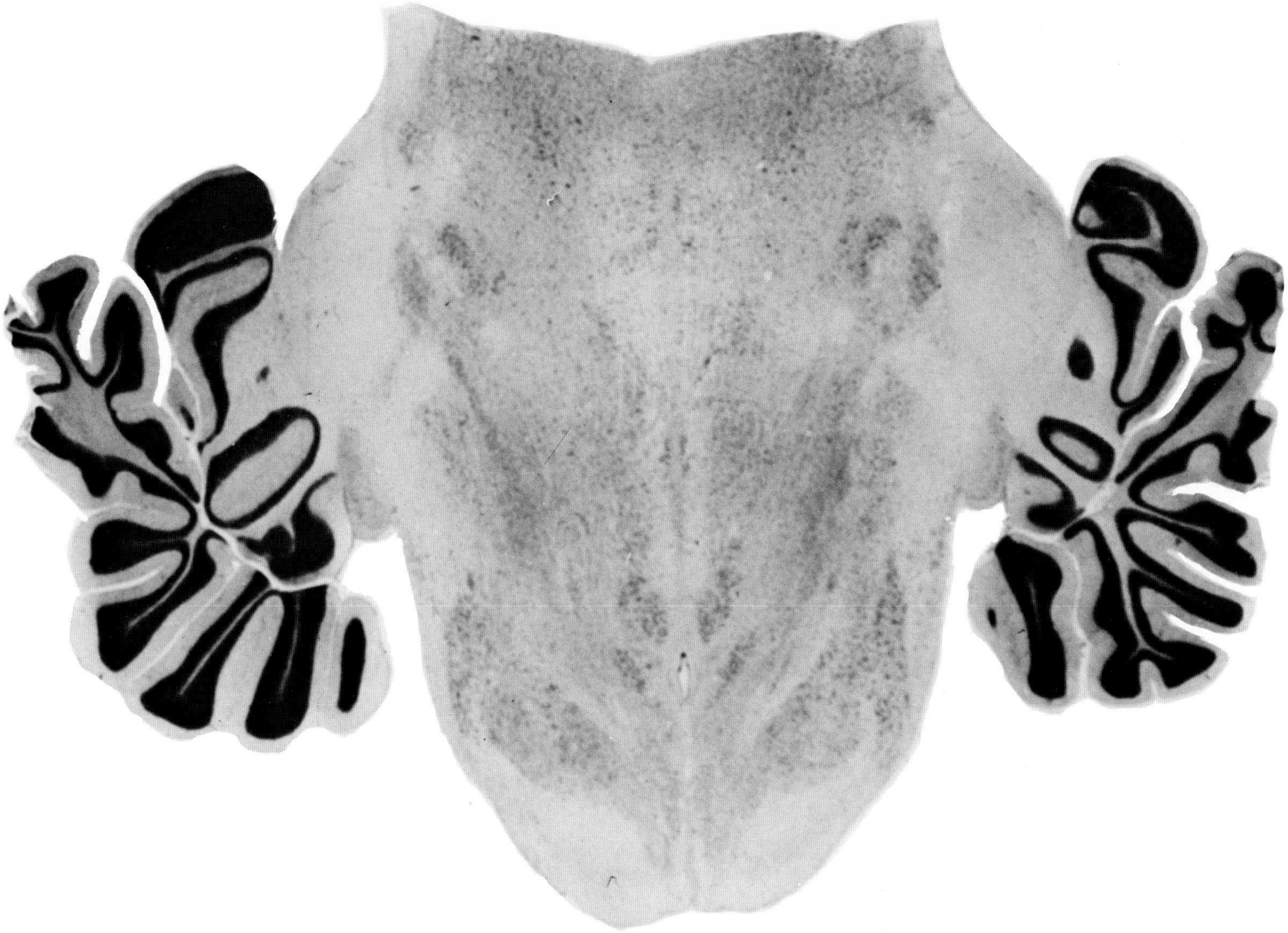

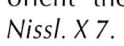

Figs. 69–70 The dorsal paraflocculus can be seen in almost its entire extent in this section ventral to the hemispheres. Folia are numbered from one to ten, according to Larsell. The most dorsal levels of the flocculus have come into view medial to the dorsal paraflocculus. As noted in the Introduction and in the Sagittal Series, the numbering of folia is less definitive for the flocculus but is presented to orient the reader from one section to the next. *Nissl. X 7.*

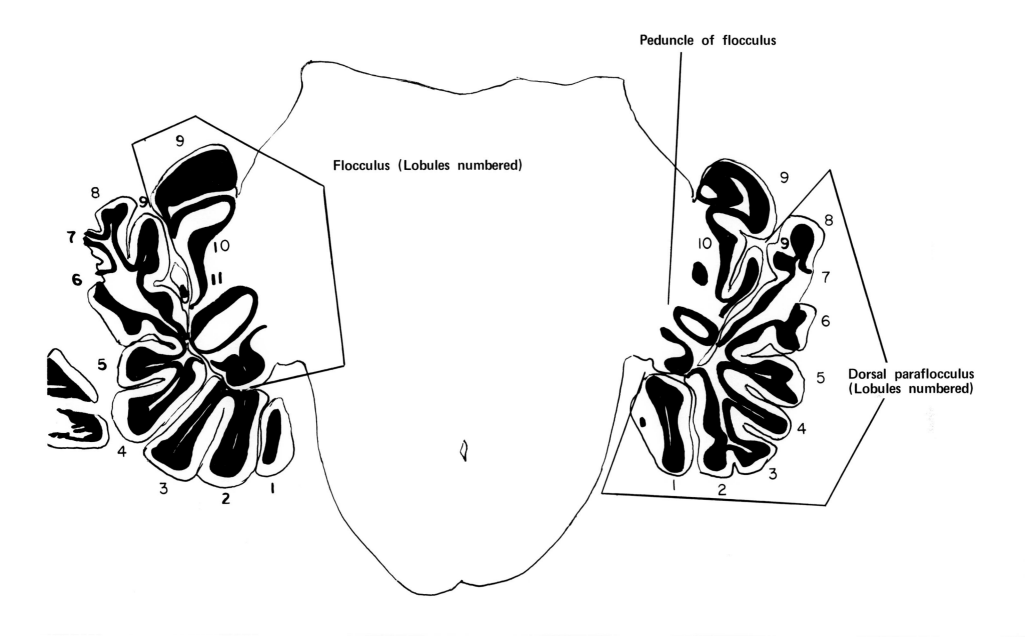

Peduncle of flocculus

Flocculus (Lobules numbered)

Dorsal paraflocculus
(Lobules numbered)

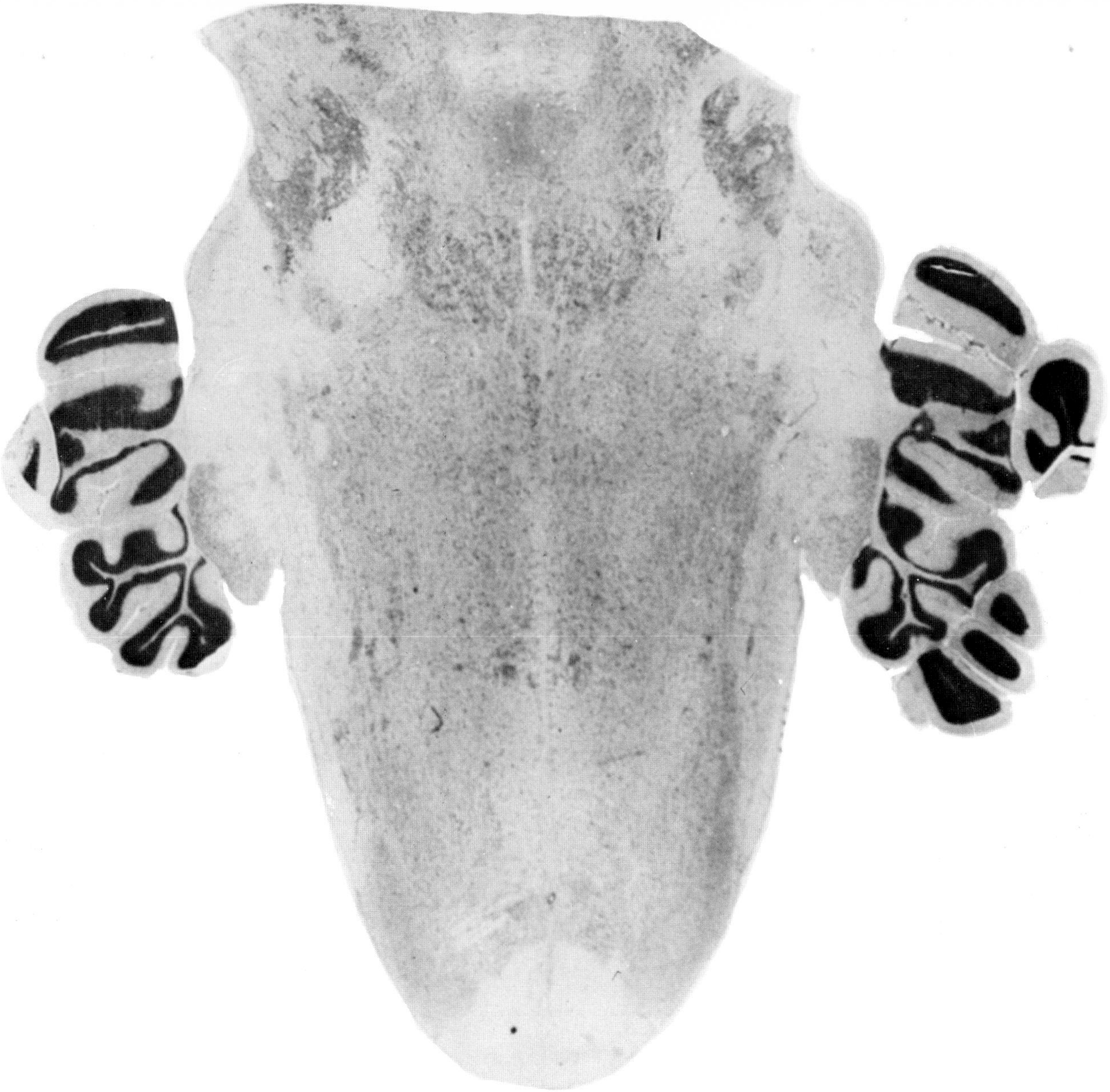

Figs. 71–72 Ventral levels of the dorsal para-flocculus are seen in this section and numbered. The folia of the flocculus are more prominent and also numbered.   *Nissl. X 8.*

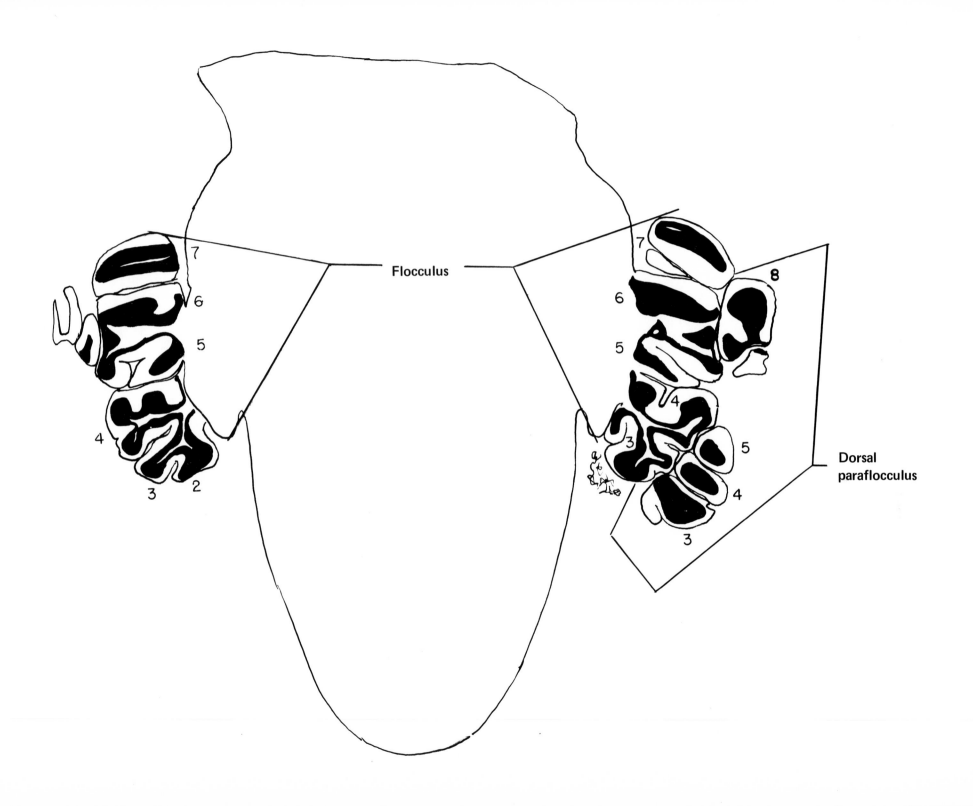

Flocculus

Dorsal
paraflocculus

89

Transverse Section Series

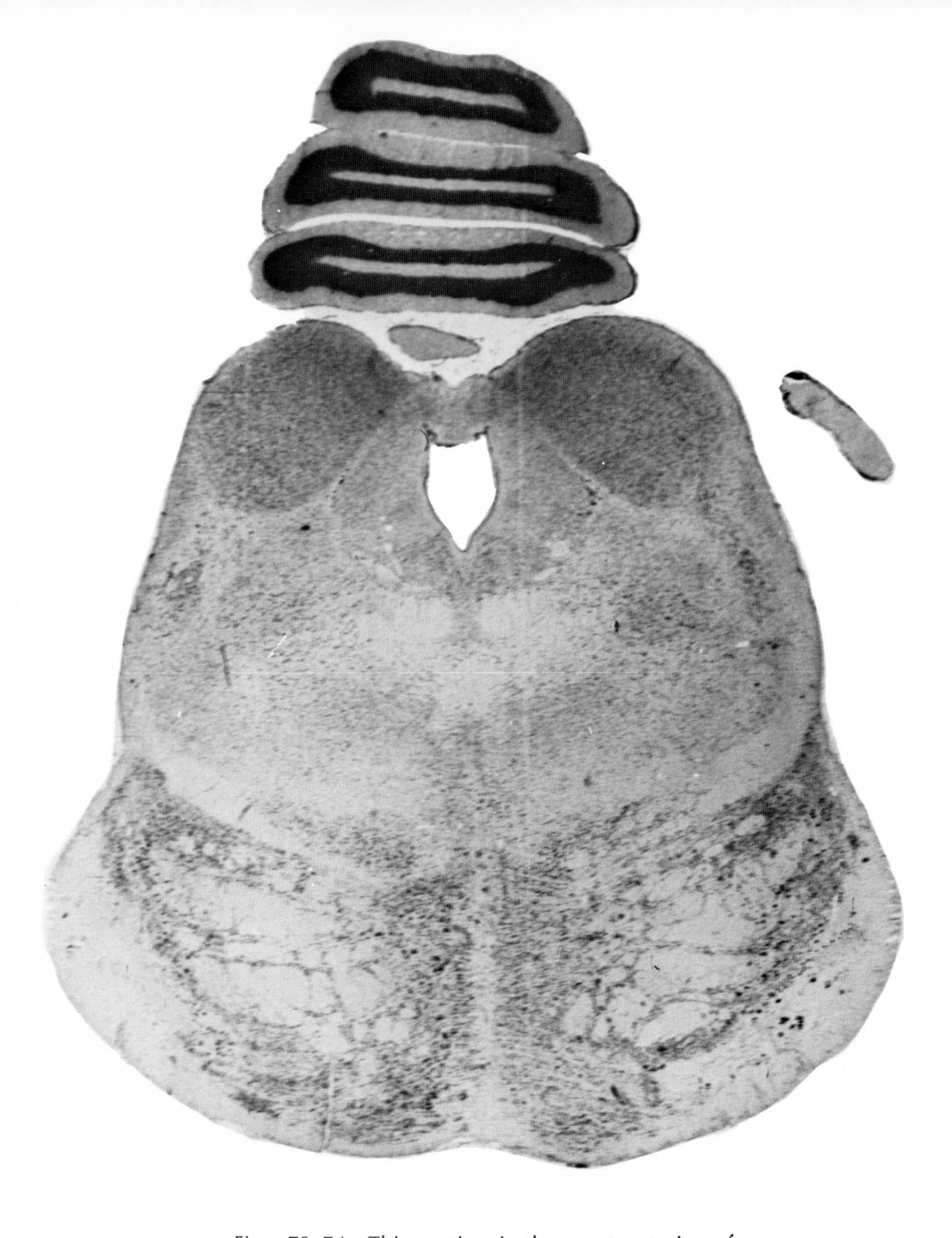

Figs. 73–74 This section is the most anterior of this series, and demonstrates the most rostral structures of the vermis, namely, laminae III_b and III_a of the central lobule.   *Nissl. X 9.*

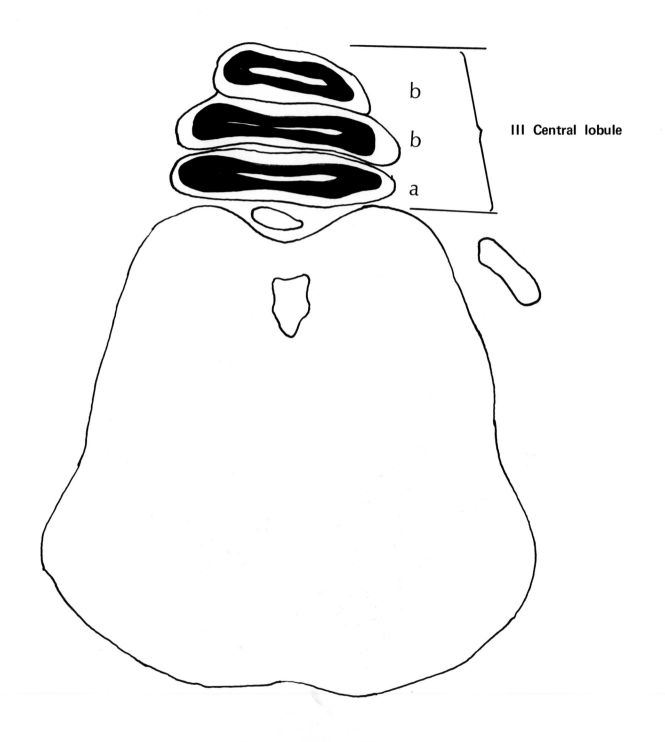

b

b

a

III Central lobule

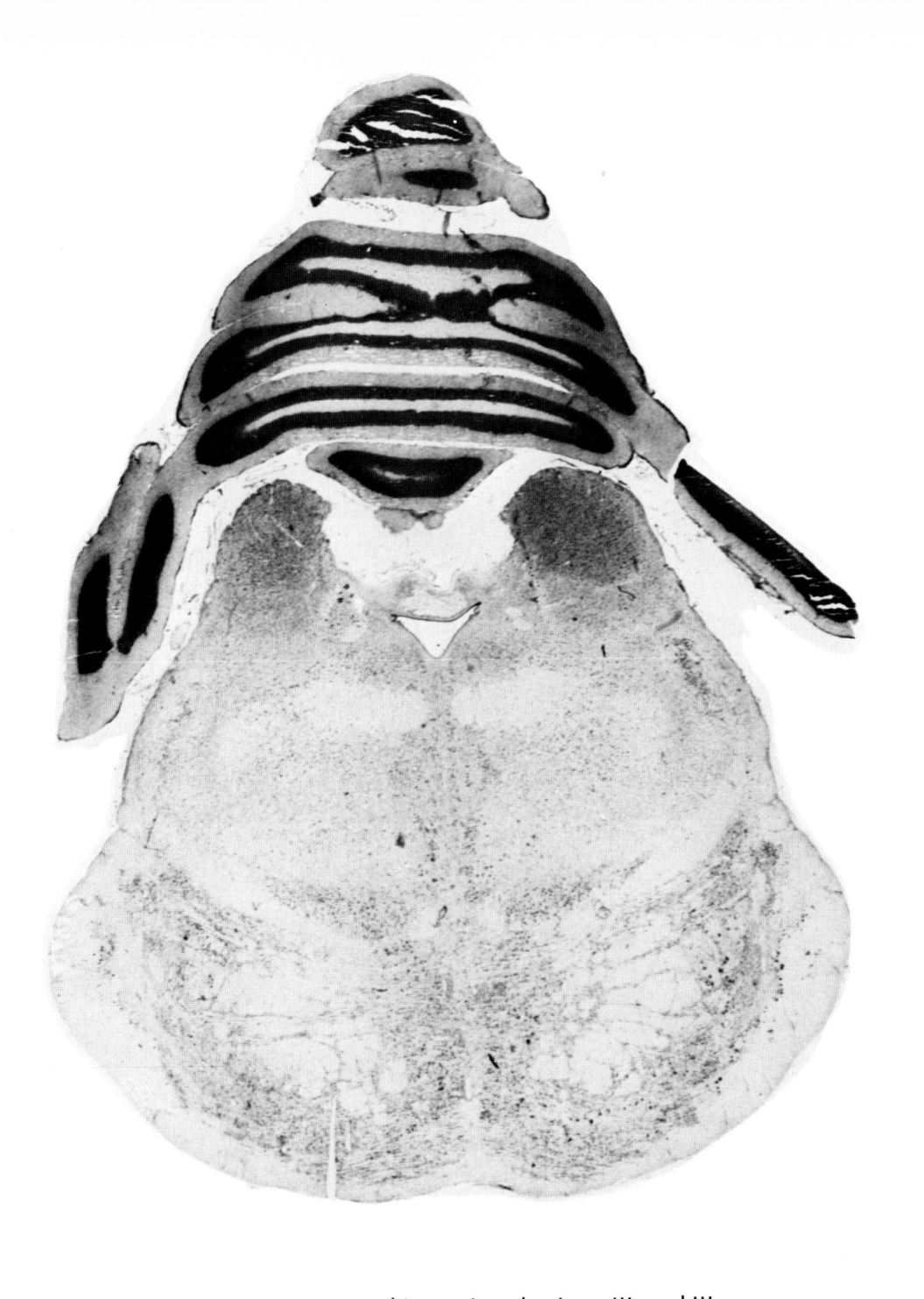

Figs. 75–76 In this section, laminae III_a and III_b of the central lobule begin to extend into the hemispheres, and lobule IV of the vermis, representing the culmen, appears dorsal to the central lobule. *Nissl. X 9.*

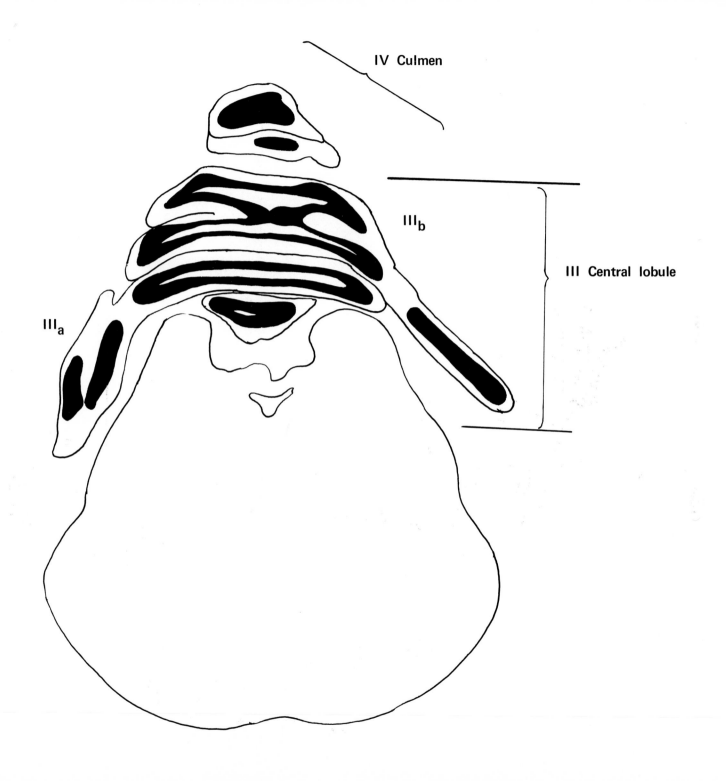

IV Culmen

III$_b$

III$_a$

III Central lobule

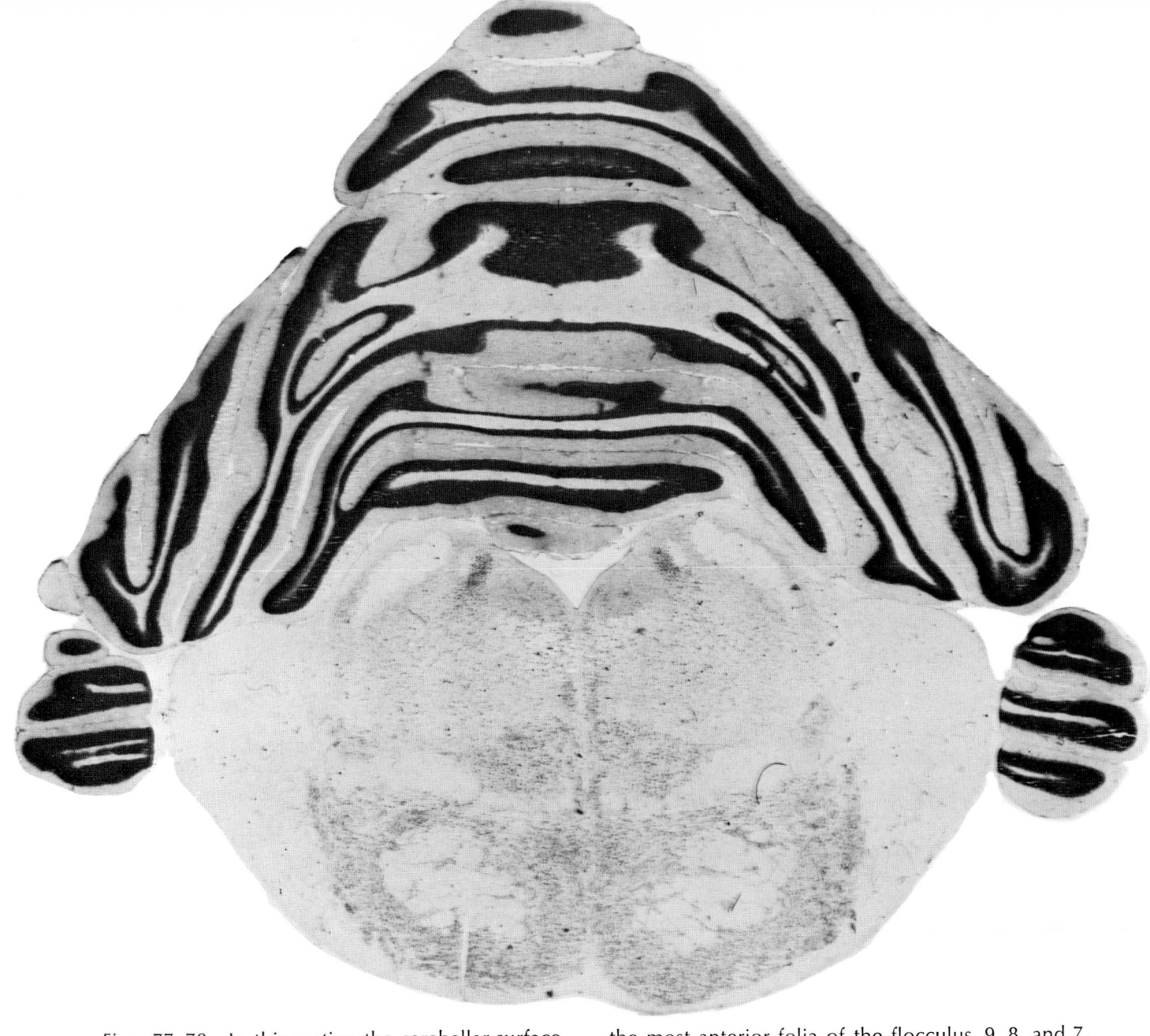

Figs. 77–78 In this section the cerebellar surface is composed almost entirely of laminae IV_a and IV_b of the anterior quadrangular lobule, the hemispheric counterpart of the vermal culmen. The central lobule no longer reaches the dorsal cerebellar surface, and consists not only of lobule III, but also of laminae II_a and II_b, newly appearing in this section. Also present for the first time in this section are the most anterior folia of the flocculus, 9, 8, and 7, visible ventrolaterally.

The folia of the flocculus are numbered consecutively from 1 (ventrocaudal) to 10 (dorsorostral), as described in the Introduction (p. 12). This numbering is less definitive than for the folia of the dorsal paraflocculus, and is presented mainly to orient the reader in moving from one section to the next. *Nissl. X 9.*

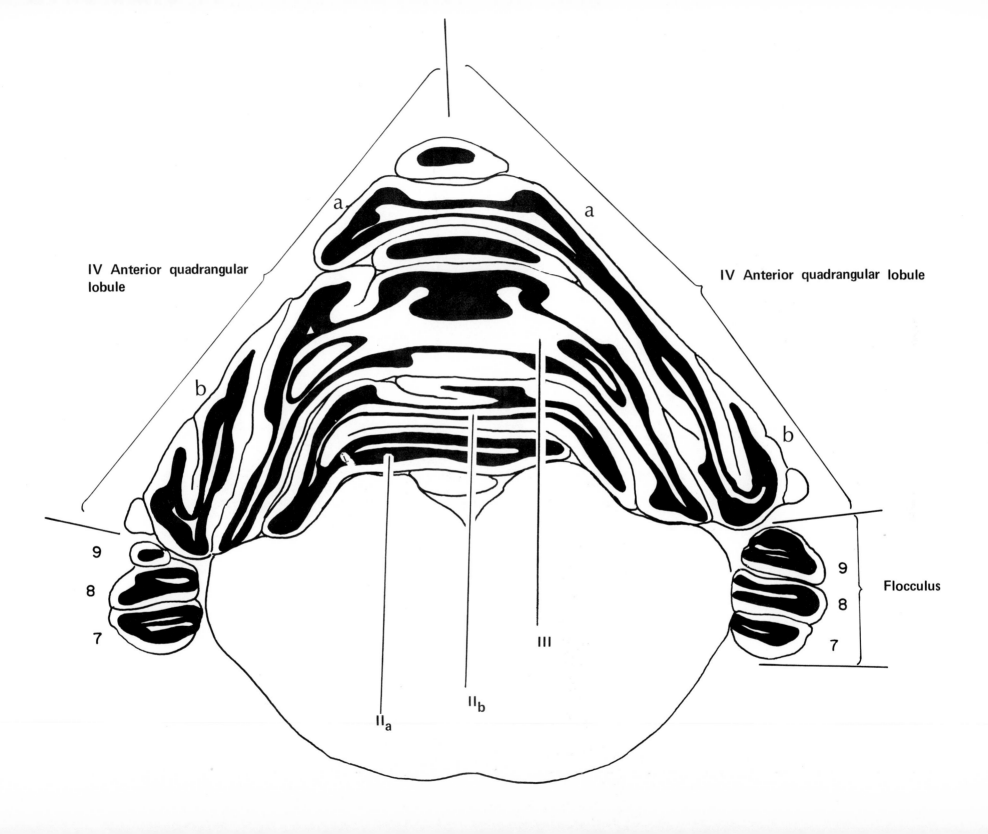

IV Anterior quadrangular lobule

IV Anterior quadrangular lobule

Flocculus

a

a

b

b

9

8

7

9

8

7

II_a

II_b

III

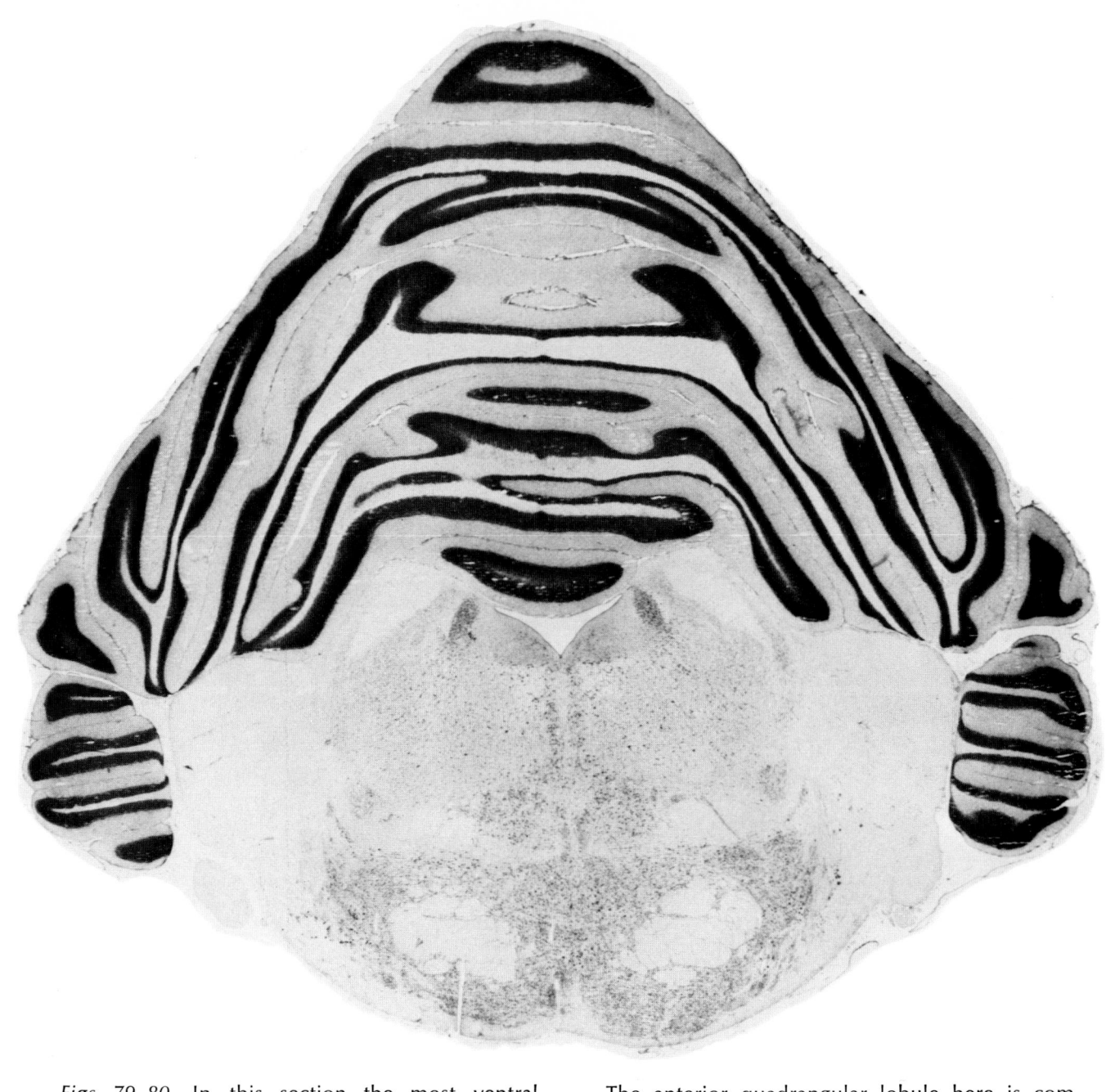

Figs. 79–80 In this section the most ventral structure of the anterior cerebellum, the lingula, appears as lamina I_{b-c}. The central lobule, present in the interior, is composed of lobule III, and of laminae II_a and II_b, which are merging into a common core.

The anterior quadrangular lobule here is composed chiefly of laminae **a** and **b** of lobule IV, but laterally small parts of lobule V can be seen. Folia 9, 8, and 7 of the flocculus are present bilaterally, unchanged from the previous section, and folium 6 of the flocculus is seen on the left.   *Nissl. X 8.*

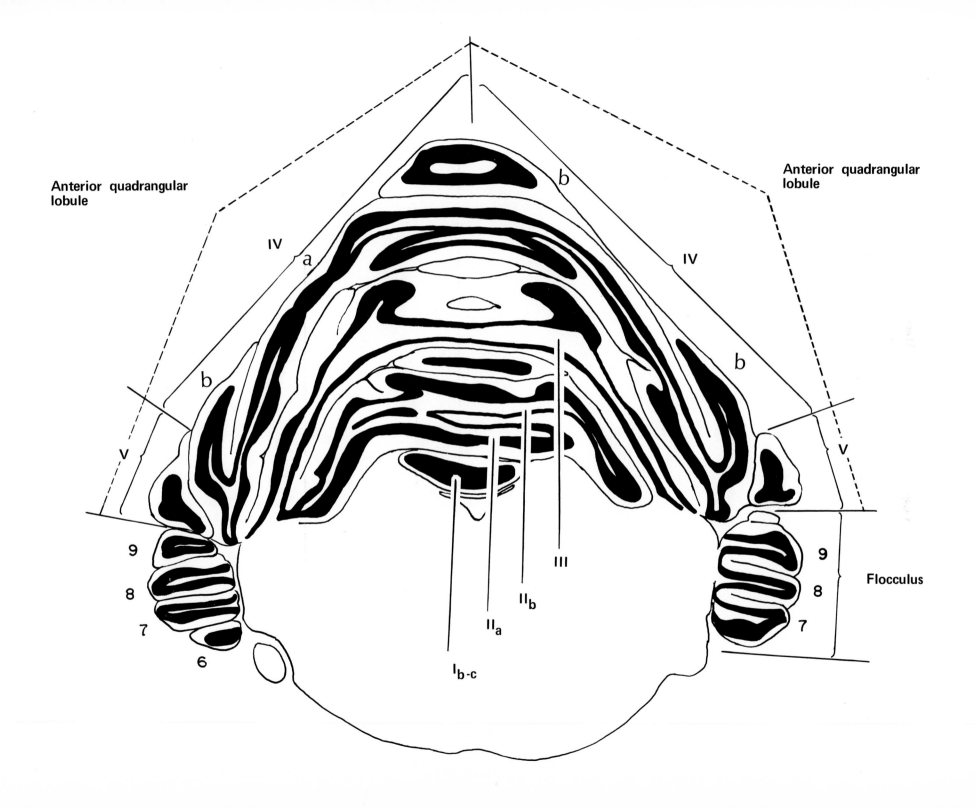

b

IV

IV

a

b

b

V

V

9

8

7

6

III

II_b

II_a

I_b-c

9

8

7

Flocculus

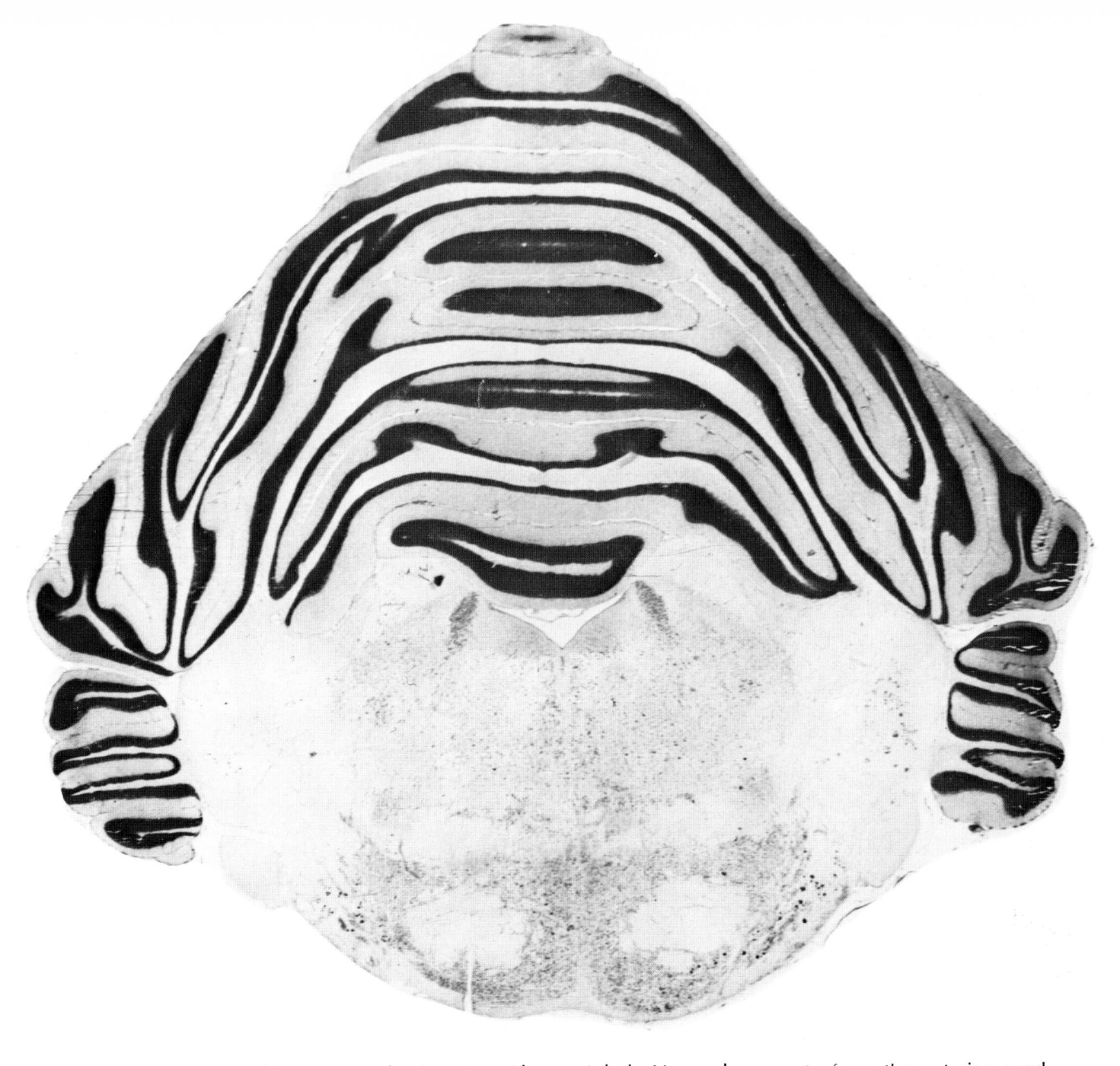

Figs. 81–82 In this section lamina I$_{b-c}$ (the lingula) is unchanged. In the central lobule, lobule III is unchanged, while laminae **a** and **b** of lobule II have merged into a single core (II$_{a-b}$).

Laminae **a** and **b** of lobule IV, and portions of lobule V, can be seen to form the anterior quadrangular lobule.

In the flocculus, folia 10, 9, 8, and 7 are visible on the right, while folia 9, 8, 7, and 6 are present on the left. *Nissl. X 8.*

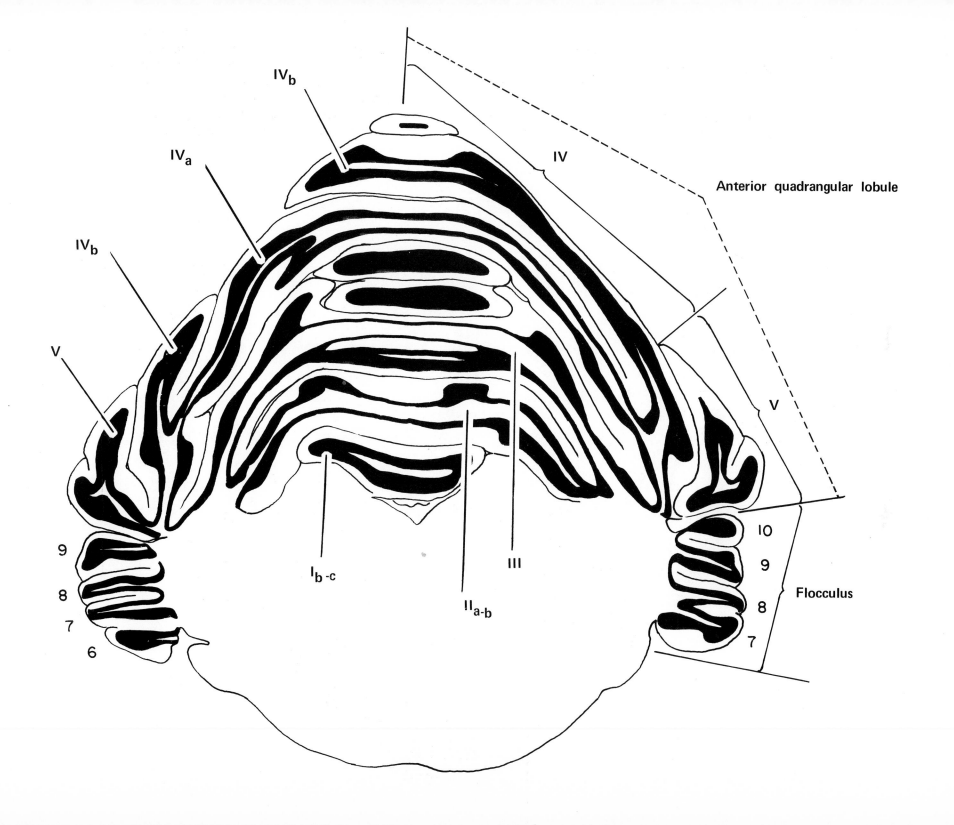

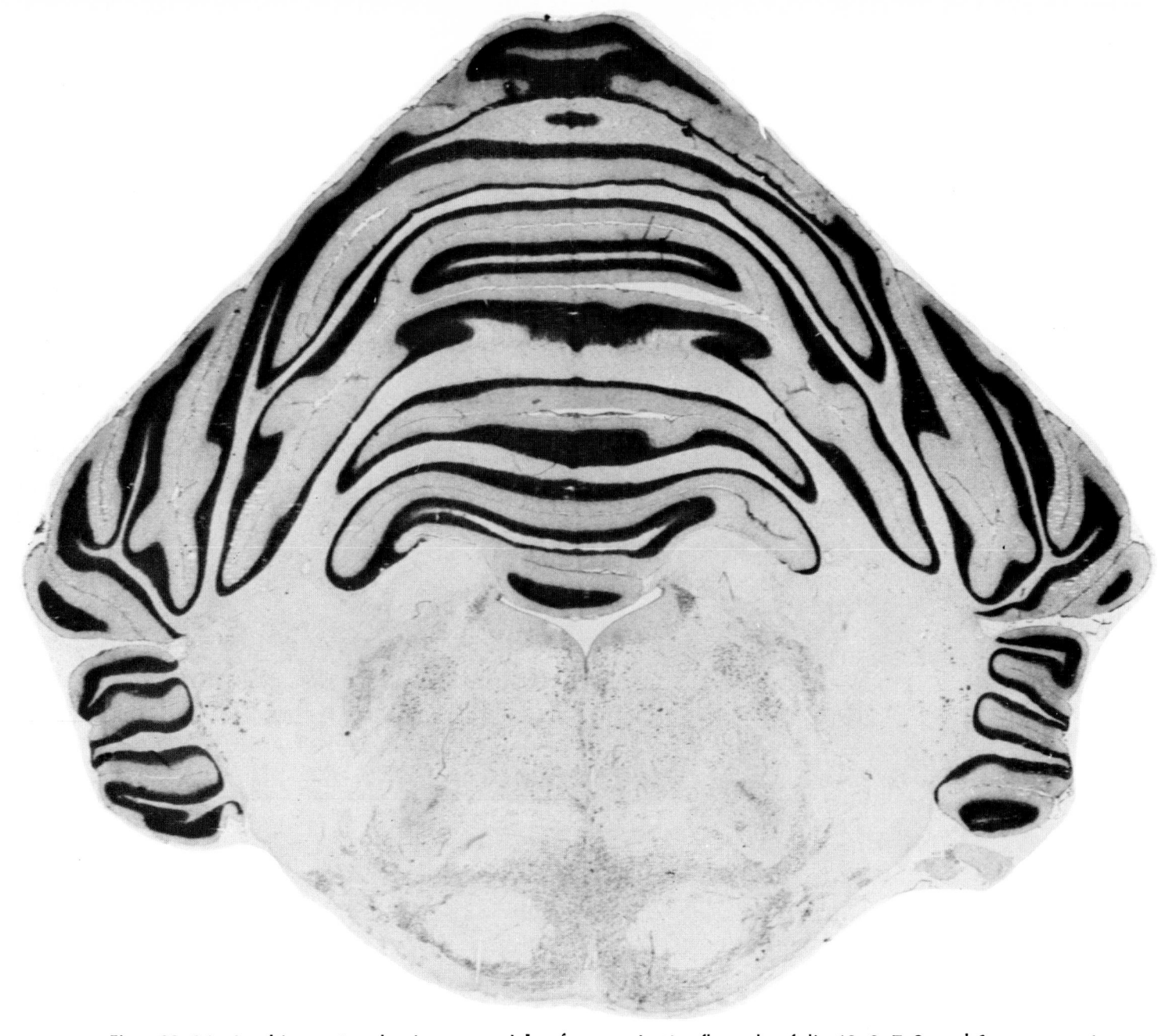

Figs. 83–84 In this section laminae **a** and **b** of lobule V form a significant part of the anterior quadrangular lobule as do laminae **a** and **b** of lobule IV. Only the cores of lobules II and III remain of the central lobule. The lingula here is composed not only of laminae I$_{b-c}$, but also of folium I$_{a}$, visible ventrally.

In the flocculus folia 10, 9, 7–8, and 6 are present on the right, and folia 9, 7–8, and 6 are present on the left.

The most anterior extent of the simple lobule is visible ventrolateral to the anterior quadrangular lobule.   *Nissl. X 8.*

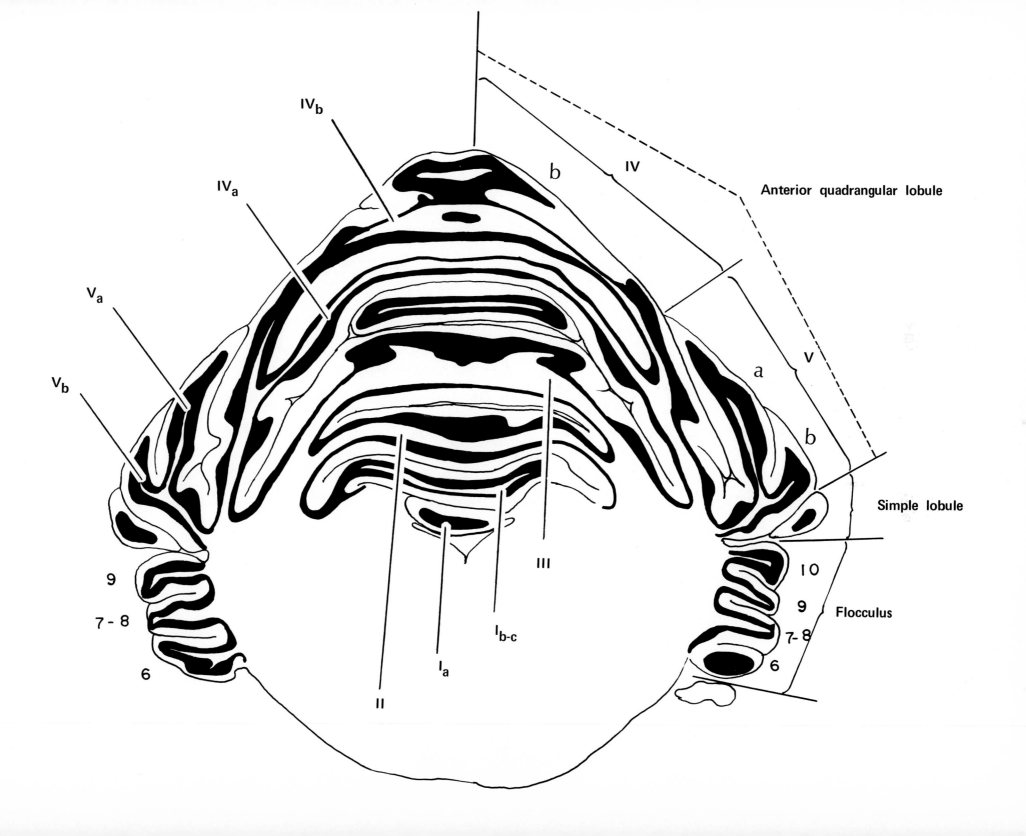

IV_b

IV_a

V_a

V_b

b

IV

Anterior quadrangular lobule

a

V

b

Simple lobule

III

I_{b-c}

I_a

II

9

7 - 8

6

10

9

Flocculus

7 - 8

6

103

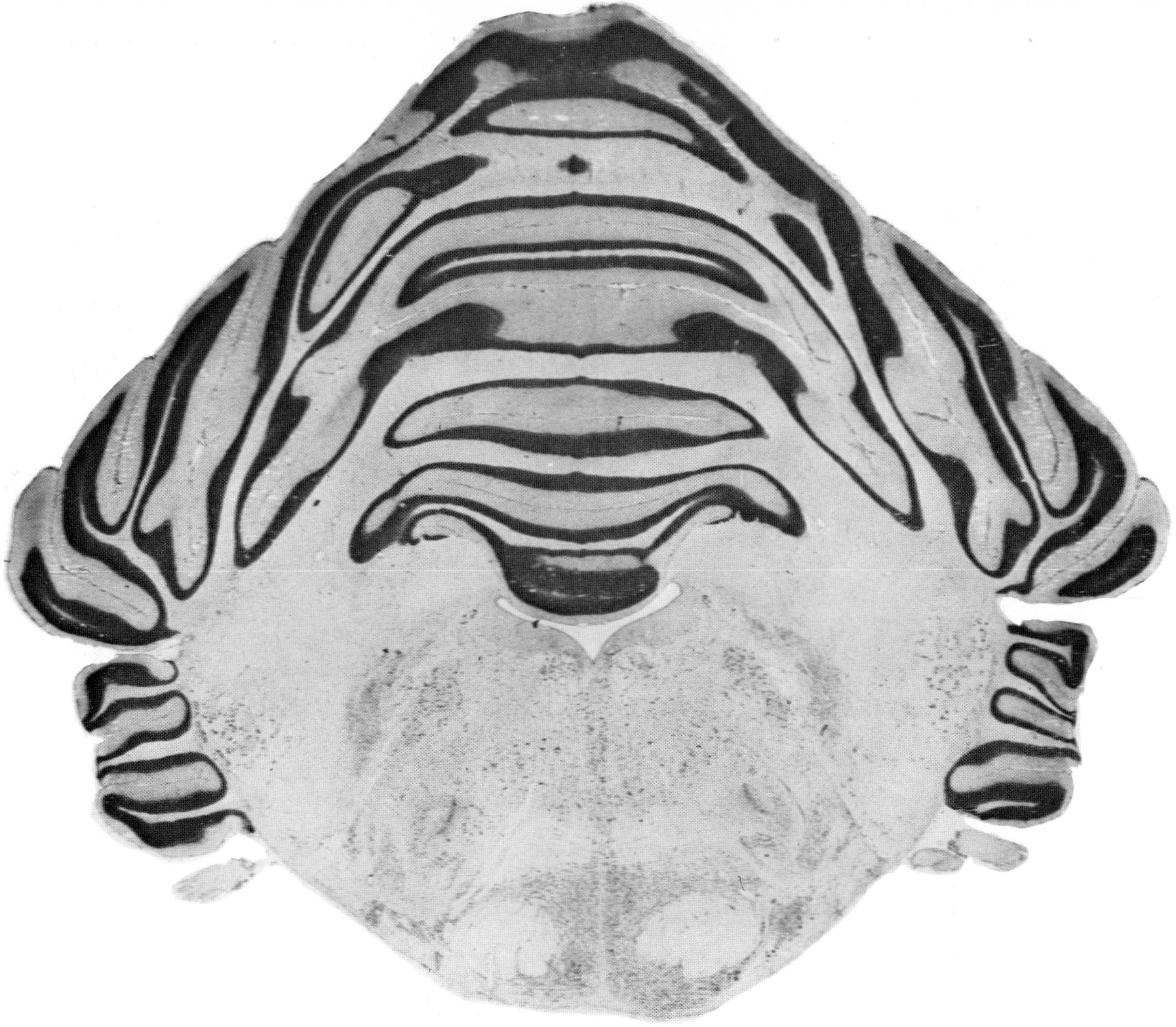

Figs. 85–86 In this section, laminae V_a, V_b, IV_a, and IV_b are unchanged from the previous section, as are the cores of lobules II and III. Folium I_a of the lingula can be seen merging into the core of laminae I_{b-c}.

The most anterior folium of the simple lobule is again present ventrolateral to the anterior quadrangular lobule.

Folia 10–6 of the flocculus are visible on both sides. *Nissl.* X 8.

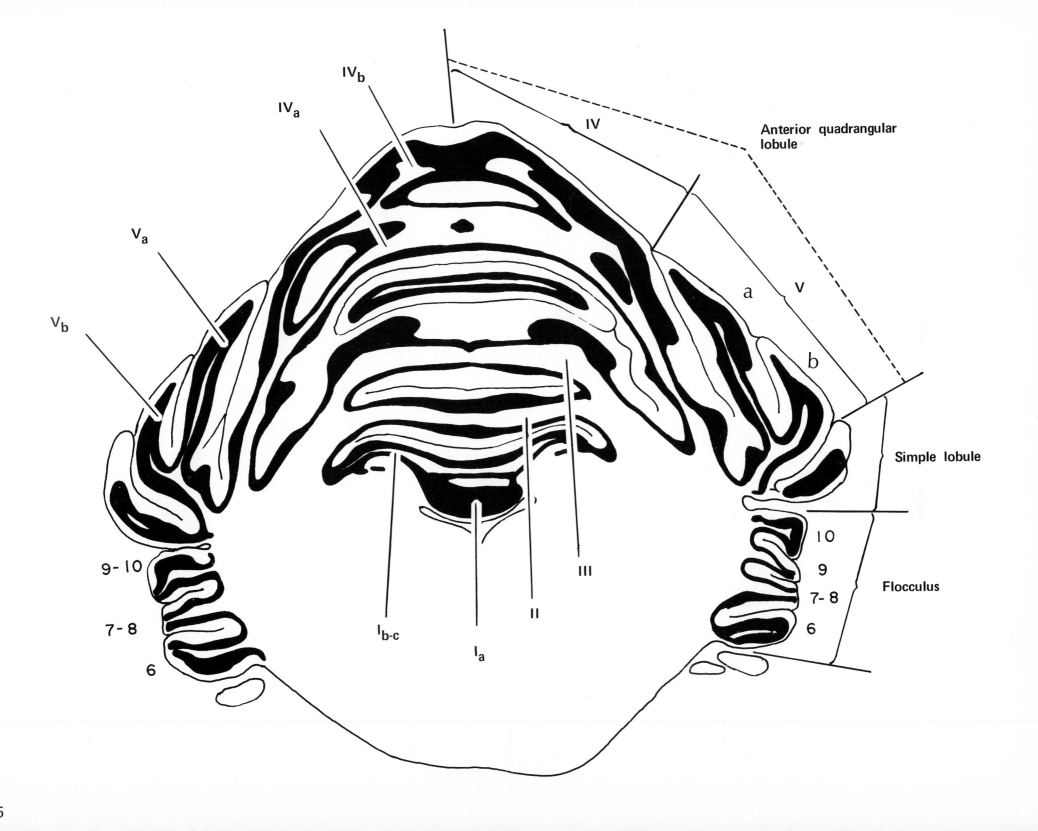

IV_b

IV_a

IV

Anterior quadrangular
lobule

V_a

V_b

a

V

b

Simple lobule

III

10

II

9

7-8

Flocculus

9-10

6

I_{b-c}

7-8

I_a

6

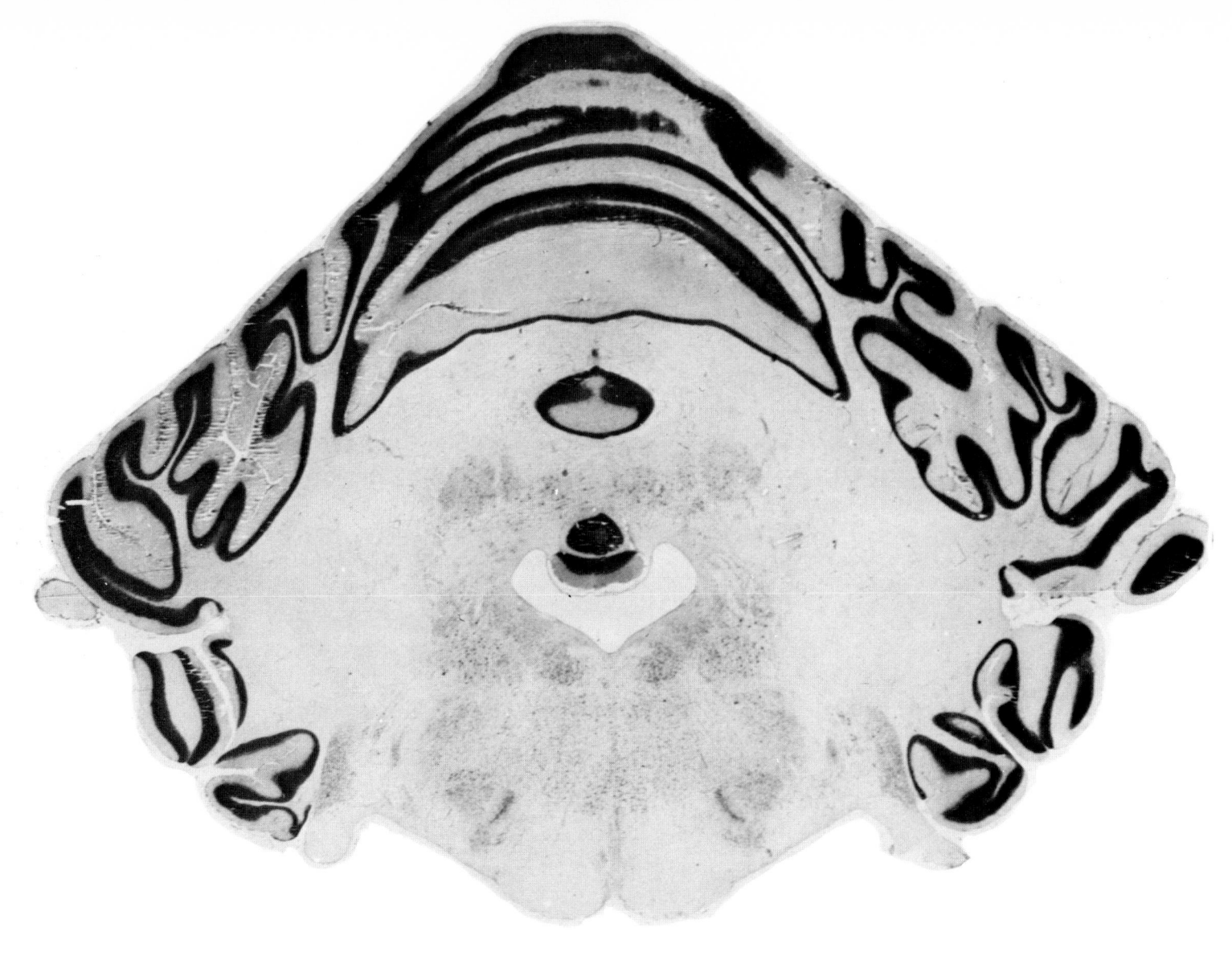

Figs. 87–88 In this section several important changes have taken place. In the anterior quadrangular lobule, laminae **a** and **b** of lobule IV are no longer present on the surface and only the core of lobule IV remains deep to lobule V, whose laminae **a** and **b** now occupy the surface. The cores of lobules II and III, and the core of lamina I$_{b-c}$, have all merged and only folium I$_a$ remains of the lingula.

The simple lobule, separated from the anterior quadrangular lobule by the primary fissure, has in-creased in size and its folia now occupy much of the lateral dorsal cerebellar surface. Folium 5 of the flocculus is present on both sides.

The dorsal paraflocculus, which lies ventral to the hemispheres and dorsolateral to the flocculus, is represented by its most rostral folium, number 10. As noted in the Introduction (p. 12), the 10 folia of the dorsal paraflocculus are numbered consecu-tively, according to Larsell (1953), from 1 (caudo-medial) to 10 (rostrolateral).   *Nissl. X 7.*

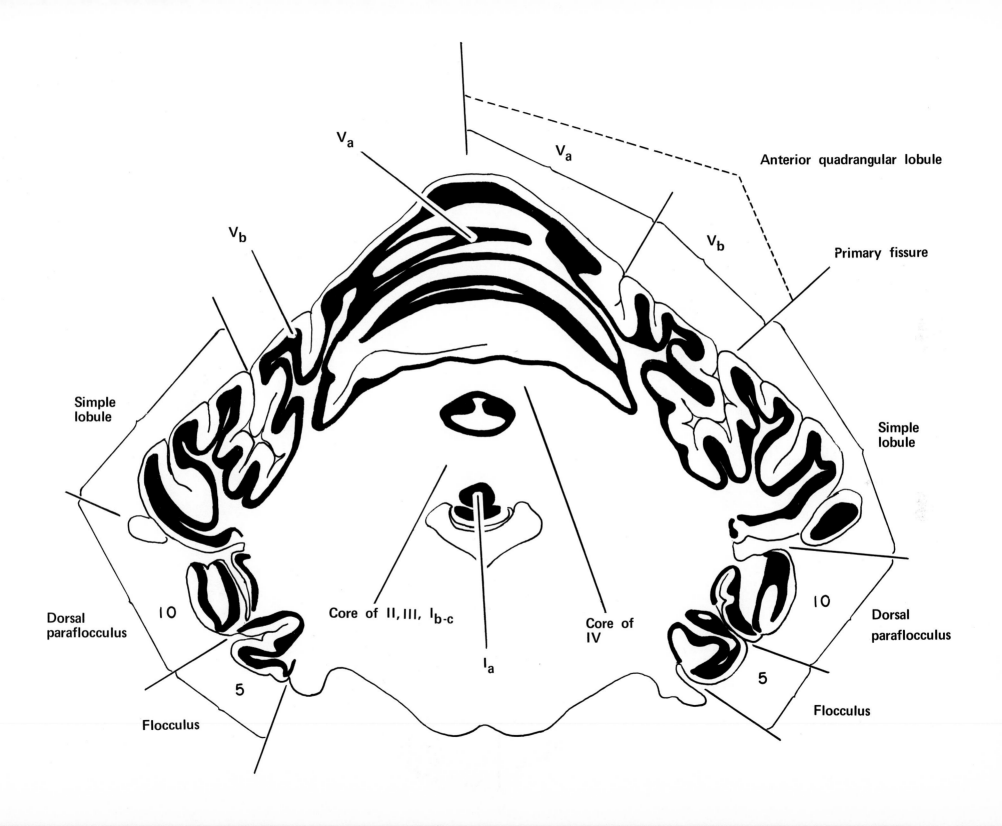

V_a

V_b

Anterior quadrangular lobule

Primary fissure

Simple lobule

Simple lobule

Dorsal paraflocculus

10

Core of II, III, I_b-c

Core of IV

I_a

10

Dorsal paraflocculus

Flocculus

5

5

Flocculus

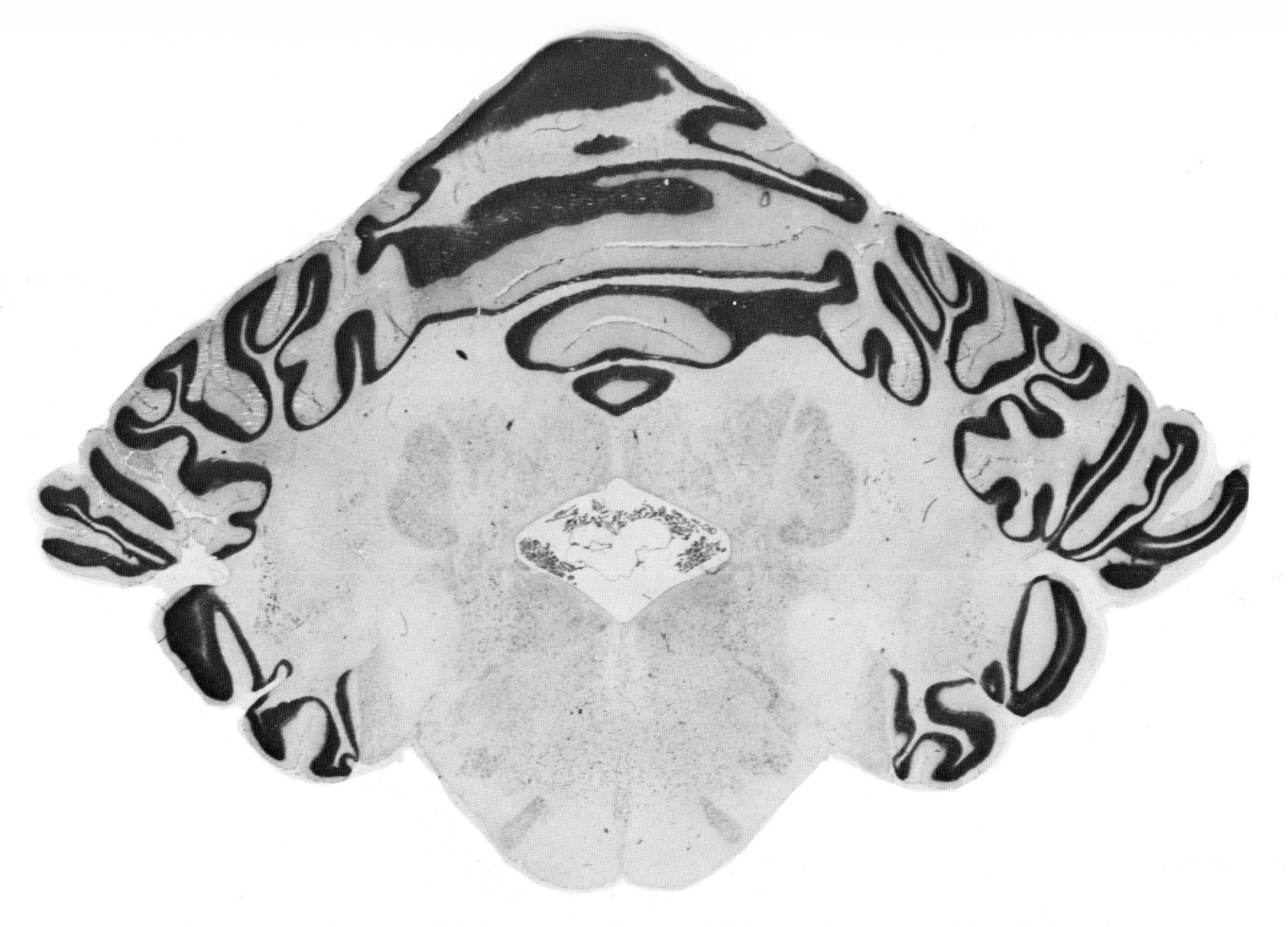

Figs. 89–90 In this section, lobules I, II, III, and IV are merged into a single core. Lobule V, with its two laminae, V_a and V_b, makes up the anterior quadrangular lobule.

The simple lobule, present laterally, is unchanged and separated from the anterior quadrangular lobule by the primary fissure.

The most anterior folia of the ansiform lobule, those of crus I, are present ventrolateral to the simple lobule, and are separated from the latter by the posterior superior fissure.

The fourth ventricle can be seen separating the central medullary core of the cerebellum from the brain stem.

Folia 5 and 4 of the flocculus are present on both sides, as is folium 10 of the dorsal paraflocculus. *Nissl. X 7.*

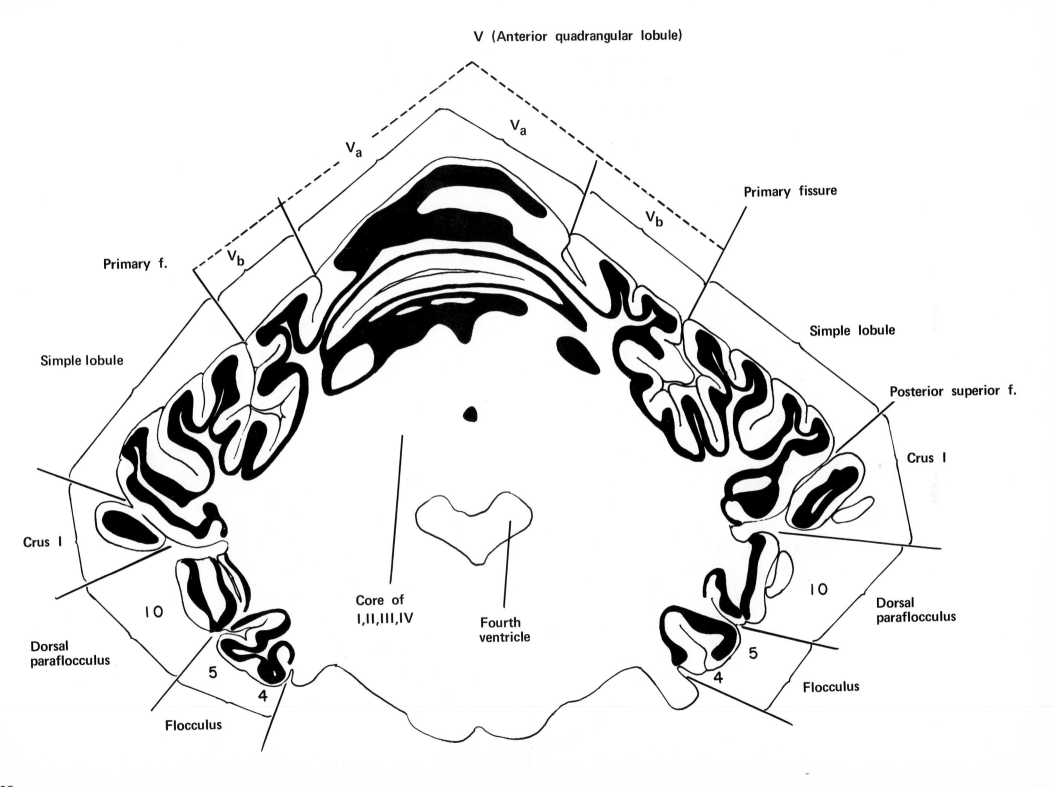

V (Anterior quadrangular lobule)

V_a

V_a

Primary fissure

V_b

Primary f.

V_b

Simple lobule

Simple lobule

Posterior superior f.

Crus I

Crus I

10

10

Dorsal paraflocculus

Core of I, II, III, IV

Dorsal paraflocculus

Fourth ventricle

5

5

4

Flocculus

4

Flocculus

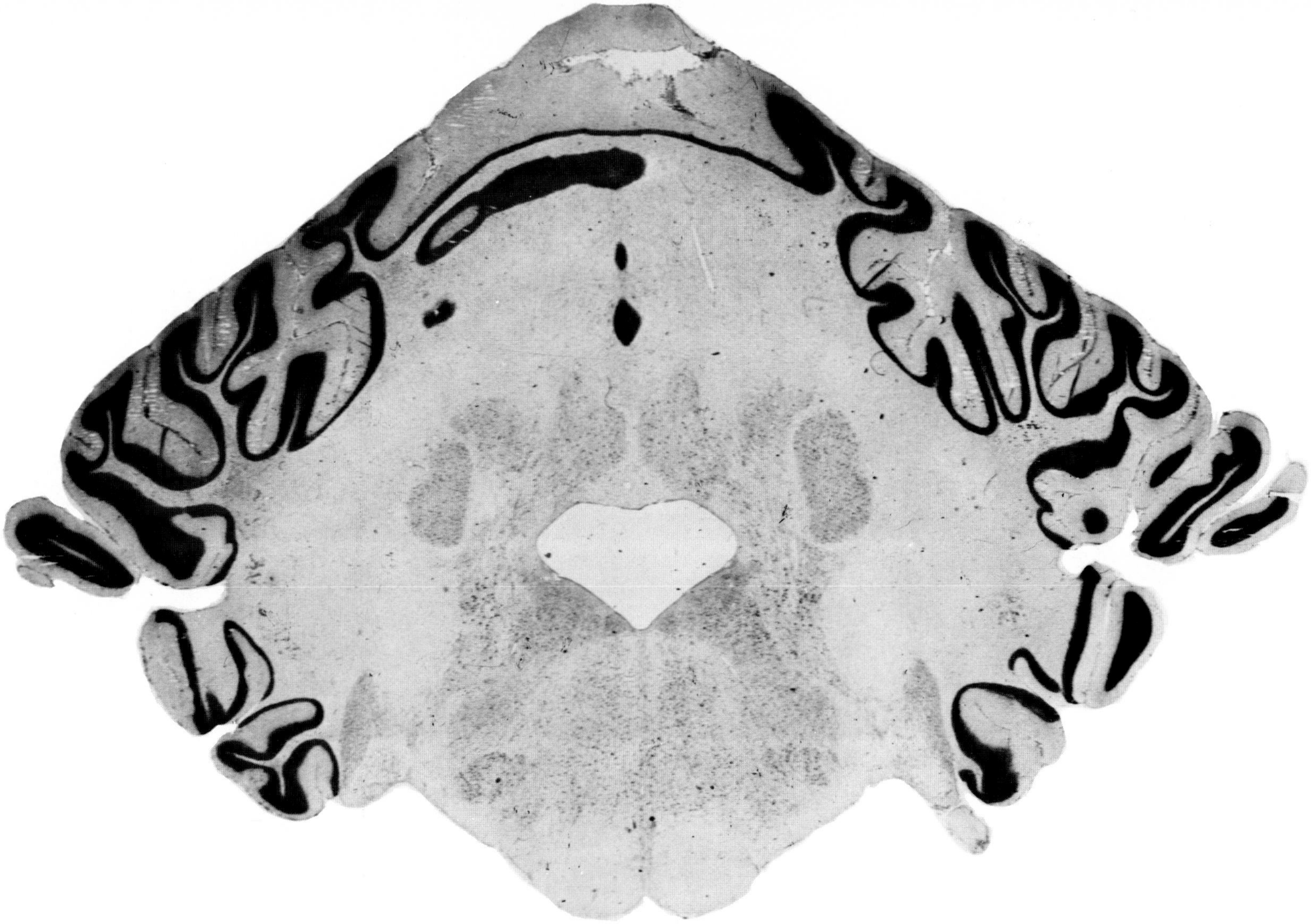

Figs. 91–92 In this section only a trace of lamina V_a is present on the cerebellar surface, and its medullary core is shown merging with that of lamina V_b, which forms most of what remains of the anterior quadrangular lobule.

The simple lobule is unchanged, as are the anterior folia of crus I.

Folia 5 and 4 of the flocculus and folium 10 of the dorsal paraflocculus are present bilaterally, as in the previous section. *Nissl. X 7.*

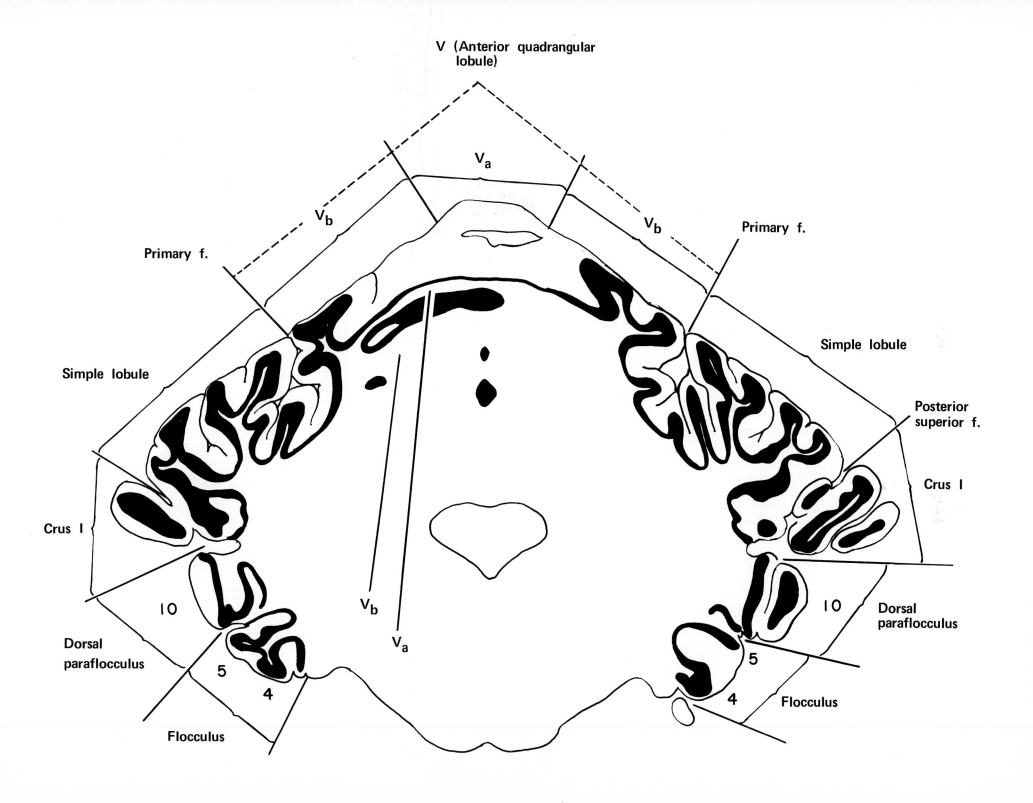

V (Anterior quadrangular lobule)

V_a

V_b

V_b

Primary f.

Primary f.

Simple lobule

Simple lobule

Posterior superior f.

Crus I

Crus I

V_b

V_a

10

10

Dorsal paraflocculus

Dorsal paraflocculus

5

5

4

4

Flocculus

Flocculus

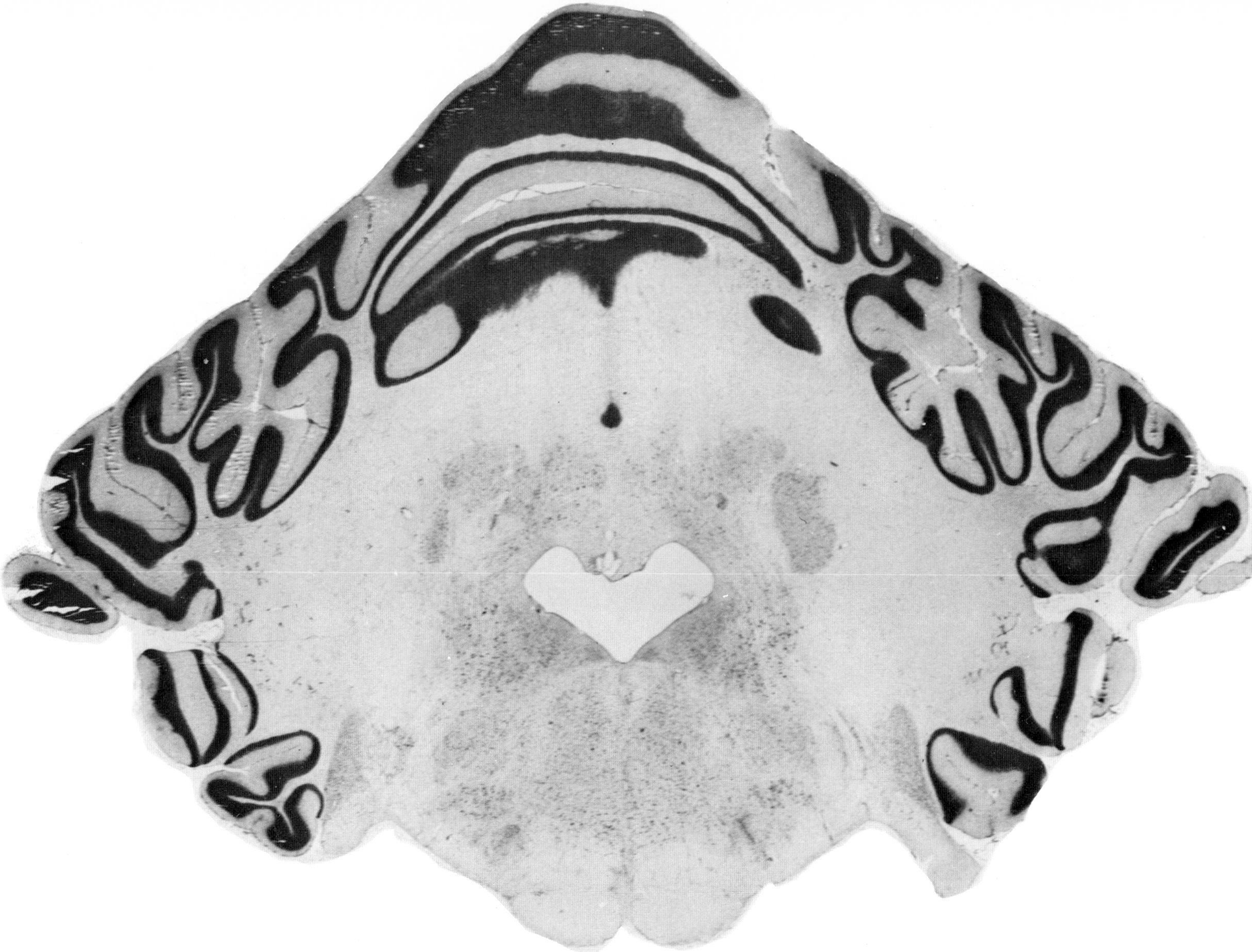

Figs. 93–94 This section passes through the most posterior lamina and folia of the anterior quadrangular lobule. Lamina V_b, and folia V_c, V_{d-e}, and V_f form the anterior bank of the primary fissure (see Figures 11–12).

The simple lobule is here more prominent. As described in the legends for Figures 25–26 and Figures 31–32, its two dorsomedial (anterior) folia are derived from vermal lobule VI, and are desig-nated VI_a and VI_{b-c}, while its two ventrolateral (posterior) folia are derived from the single vermal folium $VIIA_a$ and are designated $VIIA_a$ and $VIIA_a'$.

Crus I, separated from the simple lobule by the posterior superior fissure, is unchanged.

Folia 4 and 3 of the flocculus and folium 9 of the dorsal paraflocculus are present bilaterally. *Nissl.* X 7.

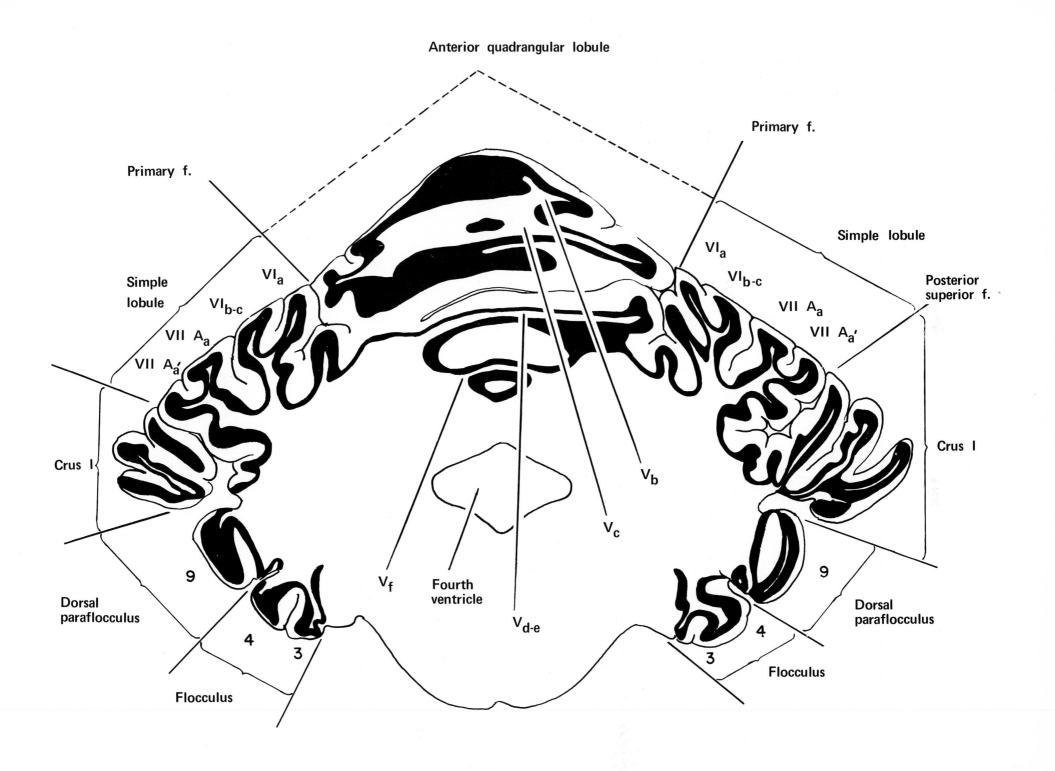

Anterior quadrangular lobule

Primary f.

Primary f.

Simple lobule

Simple lobule

VI_a

VI_{b-c}

$VII\ A_a$

$VII\ A_a'$

VI_a

VI_{b-c}

$VII\ A_a$

$VII\ A_a'$

Posterior superior f.

Crus I

Crus I

9

9

Dorsal paraflocculus

Dorsal paraflocculus

4

3

4

3

V_f

Fourth ventricle

V_{d-e}

V_c

V_b

Flocculus

Flocculus

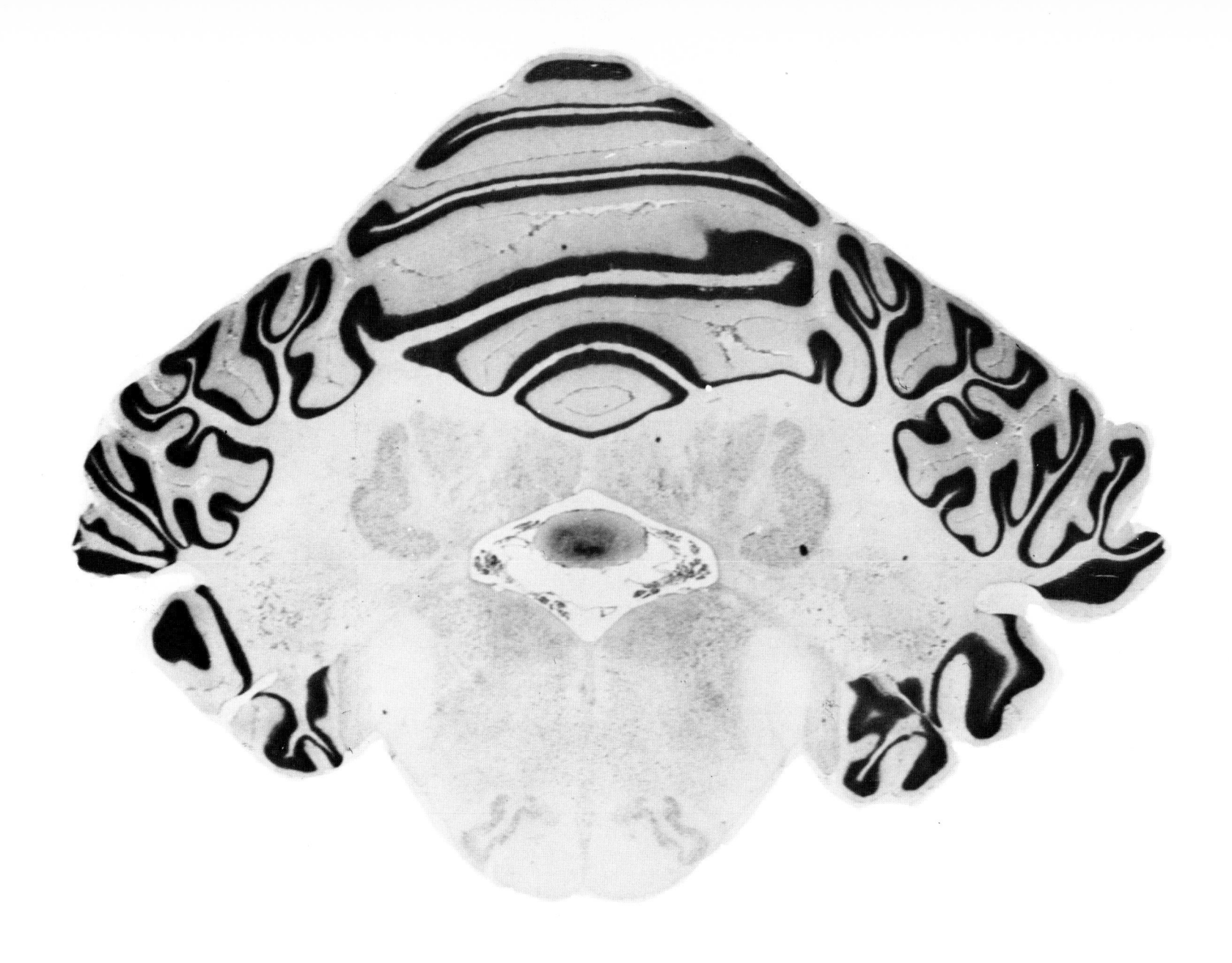

Figs. 95–96 The lamina and folia V_b, V_c, V_{d-e}, and V_f of lobule V project into the primary fissure and are unchanged.

The simple lobule with its four surface folia as described in the legend for Figures 93–94 is unchanged.

Crus I is becoming more prominent laterally, and the most rostral portion of the nodulus (**vermal lobule X**) is present near the roof of the fourth ventricle.

Folia 3 and 2 of the flocculus are present bilaterally. In the dorsal paraflocculus, folium 8 is present on the right, and folium 9 is present on the left. *Nissl. X 7.*

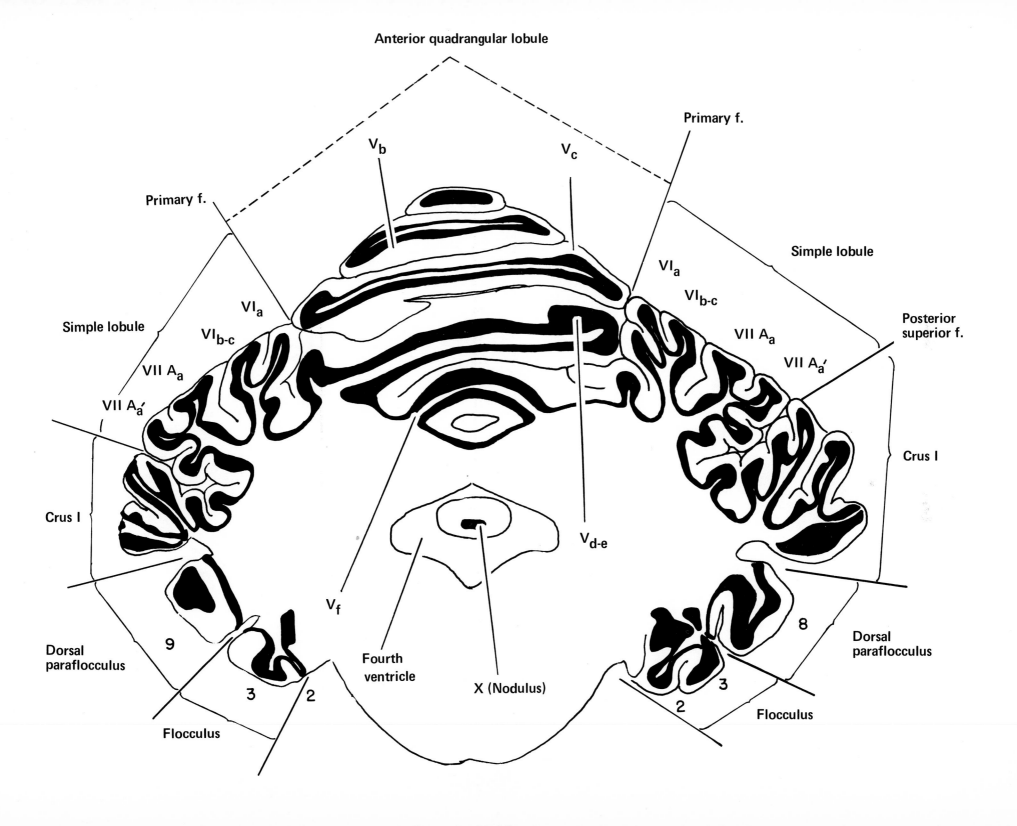

Anterior quadrangular lobule

Primary f.

V_b

V_c

Primary f.

VI_a

VI_{b-c}

Simple lobule

Simple lobule

VI_a

VI_{b-c}

$VII A_a$

$VII A_a$

$VII A_a'$

$VII A_a'$

Posterior superior f.

Crus I

Crus I

V_{d-e}

V_f

9

3

2

8

3

2

Dorsal paraflocculus

Fourth ventricle

X (Nodulus)

Dorsal paraflocculus

Flocculus

Flocculus

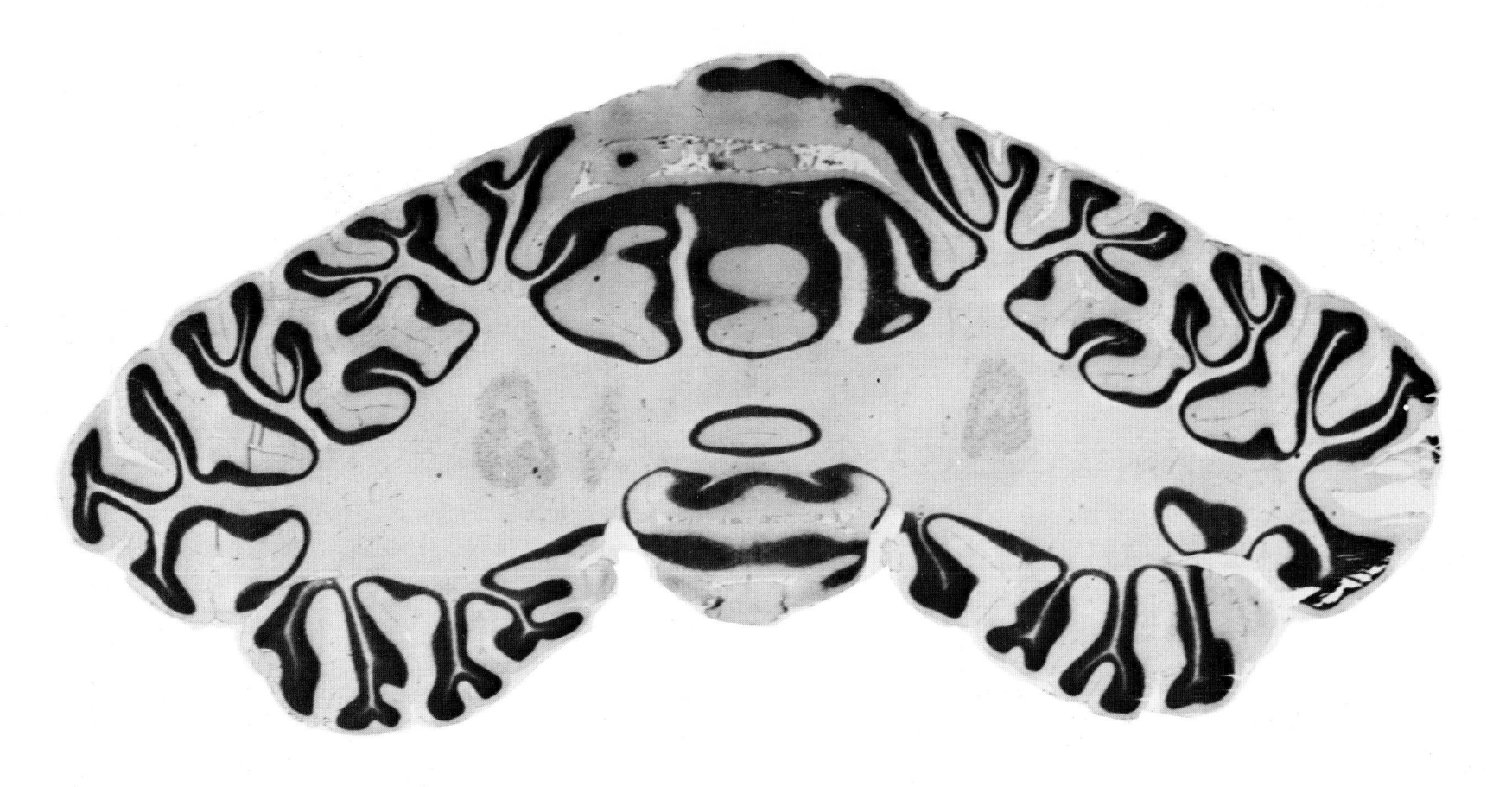

Figs. 97–98 This section passes through the posterior part of the primary fissure, and through the anterior part of the vermal portion of the simple lobule, which projects folia into the primary fissure. Vermal folium VI$_a$ is prominent medially and on the right can be seen extending laterally to form a corresponding folium in the hemispheric simple lobule. Folium VI$_{d-e}$ can be seen beneath folium VI$_a$, within the primary fissure. The other folia of the simple lobule are unchanged from the previous section.

Separated from the simple lobule by the posterior superior fissure, the ansiform lobule has become more prominent. On both sides its anterior portion, crus I, is seen, with its two subdivisions, crus I$_a$ and I$_p$, clearly separated from one another. On the right, the most rostral folium of crus II is visible ventral to crus I.

The common core of vermal lobules VI, VII, and VIII is indicated in the central medullary substance and the core of lobule IX now lies clearly separated from it.

Ventrally, the nodulus (**lobule X**) is the most prominent structure in the vermis while the dorsal paraflocculus, with its folia consecutively numbered, is the most prominent structure in the hemispheres.

The flocculus is not present at this level.   *Nissl. X 6.*

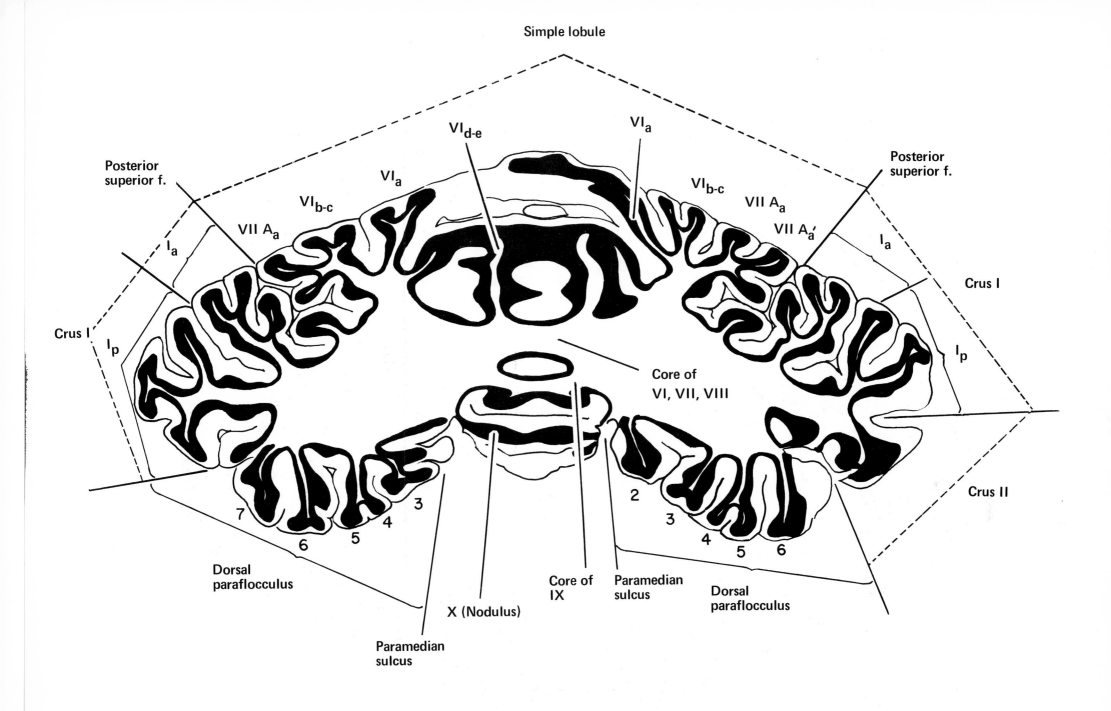

Simple lobule

Posterior superior f.

VI_{d-e}

VI_a

VI_a

Posterior superior f.

VI_{b-c}

VI_{b-c}

VII A_a

VII A_a

VII A_a'

I_a

I_a

Crus I

Crus I

I_p

I_p

Core of VI, VII, VIII

7

6

5

4

3

2

3

4

5

6

Crus II

Dorsal paraflocculus

X (Nodulus)

Core of IX

Paramedian sulcus

Dorsal paraflocculus

Paramedian sulcus

117

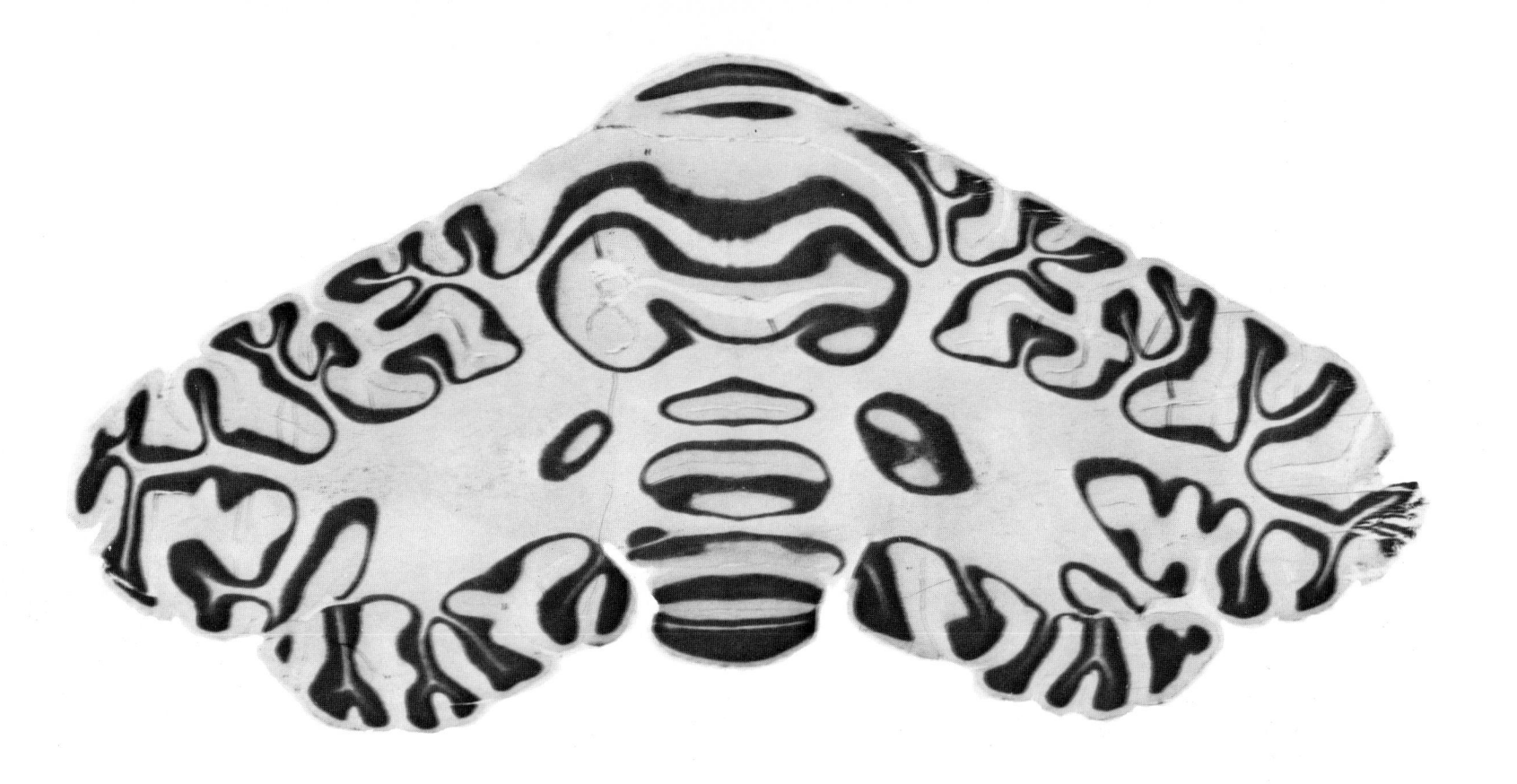

Figs. 101–102 In this section folium VI$_a$ lies within the primary fissure while folium VI$_{b-c}$ occupies the surface. Its continuity from the vermal to the hemispheric portions of the simple lobule is demonstrated.

Both crus I and crus II are prominent in the hemispheres. In the central medullary substance the core of vermal lobule VIII has now separated from the core common to lobules VI and VII, while the uvula (**lobule IX**) is present in the vermis ventrally.

The dorsal paraflocculus is present on the ventral surface of the hemispheres.   *Nissl. X 6*

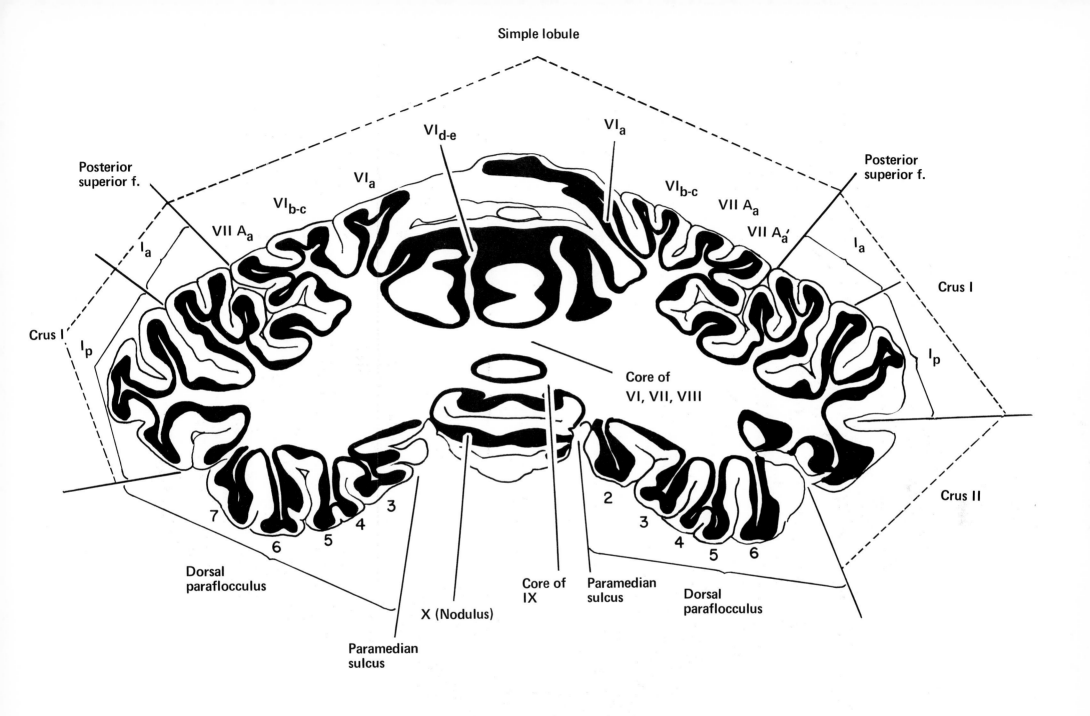

Simple lobule

Posterior superior f.

VI$_{d-e}$

VI$_a$

VI$_a$

VI$_{b-c}$

VII A$_a$

Posterior superior f.

VI$_{b-c}$

VII A$_a$

VII A$_a'$

I$_a$

Crus I

Crus I'

I$_a$

Core of VI, VII, VIII

Crus I

I$_p$

I$_p$

Core of IX

Crus II

3

2

4

3

7

4

5

6

5

6

Dorsal paraflocculus

X (Nodulus)

Core of IX

Paramedian sulcus

Dorsal paraflocculus

Paramedian sulcus

118

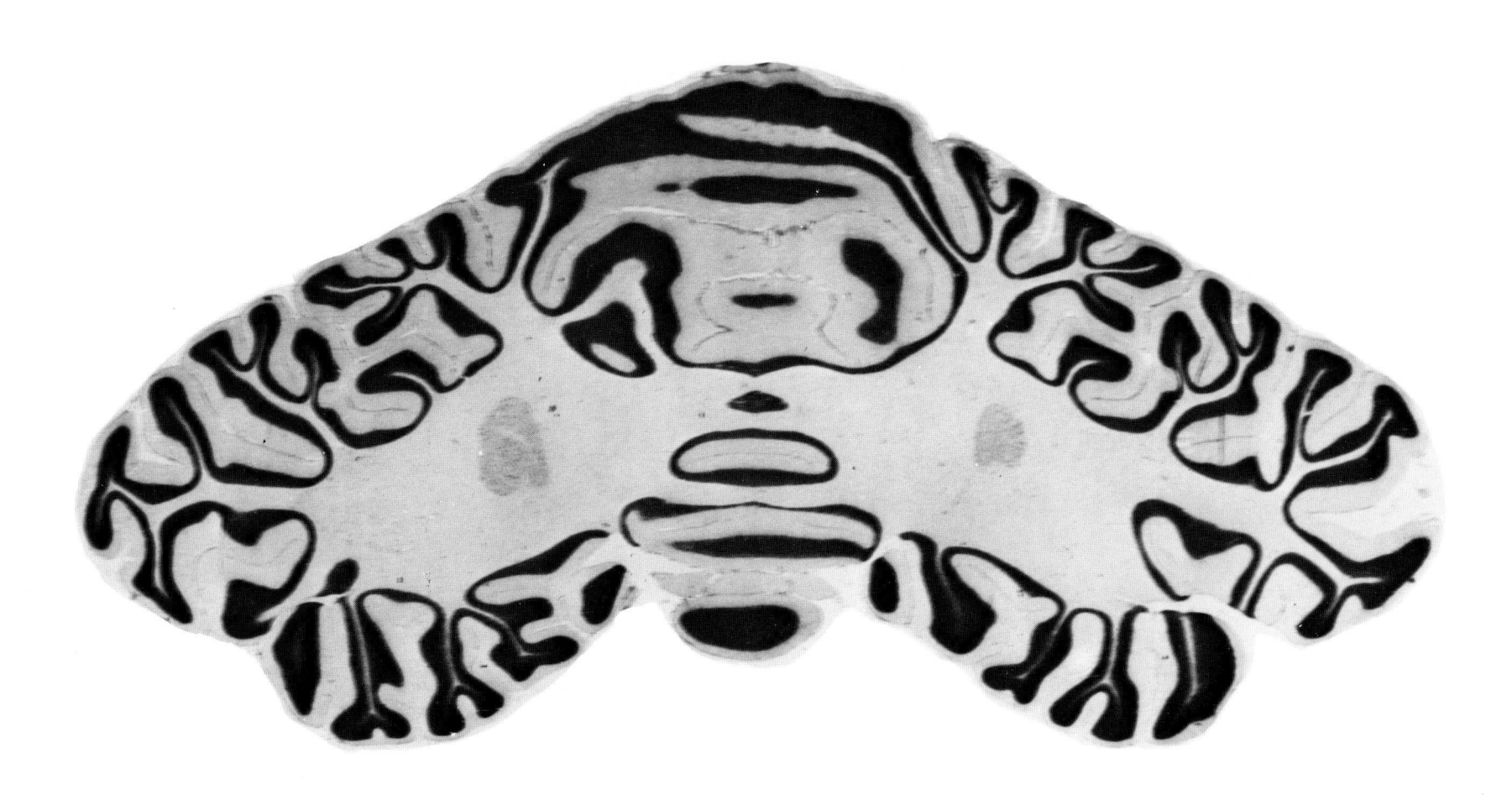

Figs. 99–100 As in the previous section, folium VIₐ of the simple lobule is prominent superiorly in the vermis, and extends bilaterally into a corresponding folium in the hemispheres. The remainder of the simple lobule is unchanged.

Crus I is more prominent laterally, and crus II, the posterior division of the ansiform lobule, can now be seen on both sides ventral to crus I.

Ventrally, the nodulus (**lobule X**) has been re-placed by the uvula (**lobule IX**) in the vermis, while the numbered folia of the dorsal paraflocculus are prominent in the hemispheres. The paramedian sulcus, which separates the vermis from the hemispheres in the posterior cerebellum, is indicated ventrally.

Again the core of lobules VI, VII, and VIII is indicated in the central medullary substance. *Nissl. X 6.*

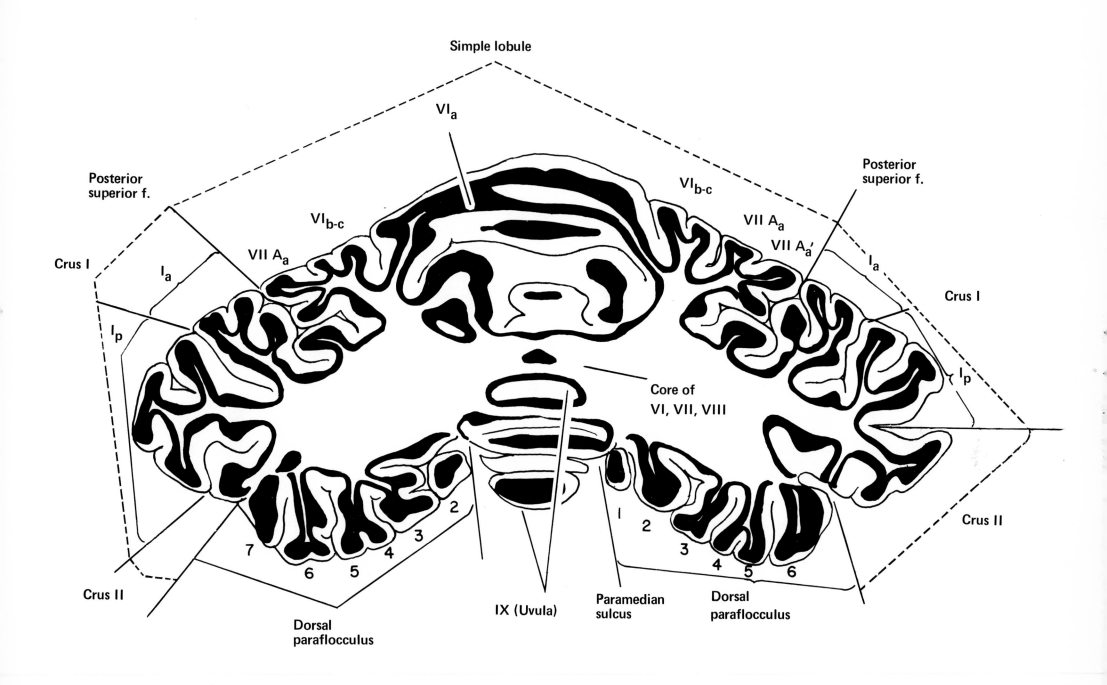

Simple lobule

VI_a

Posterior superior f.

VI_b-c

VI_b-c

VII A_a

VII A_a

VII A_a'

Crus I

I_a

I_a

Crus I

I_p

I_p

Core of
VI, VII, VIII

2

1

2

7

3

3

4

6

5

4

5

6

5

4

Crus II

IX (Uvula)

Paramedian sulcus

Dorsal paraflocculus

Crus II

Dorsal paraflocculus

Posterior superior f.

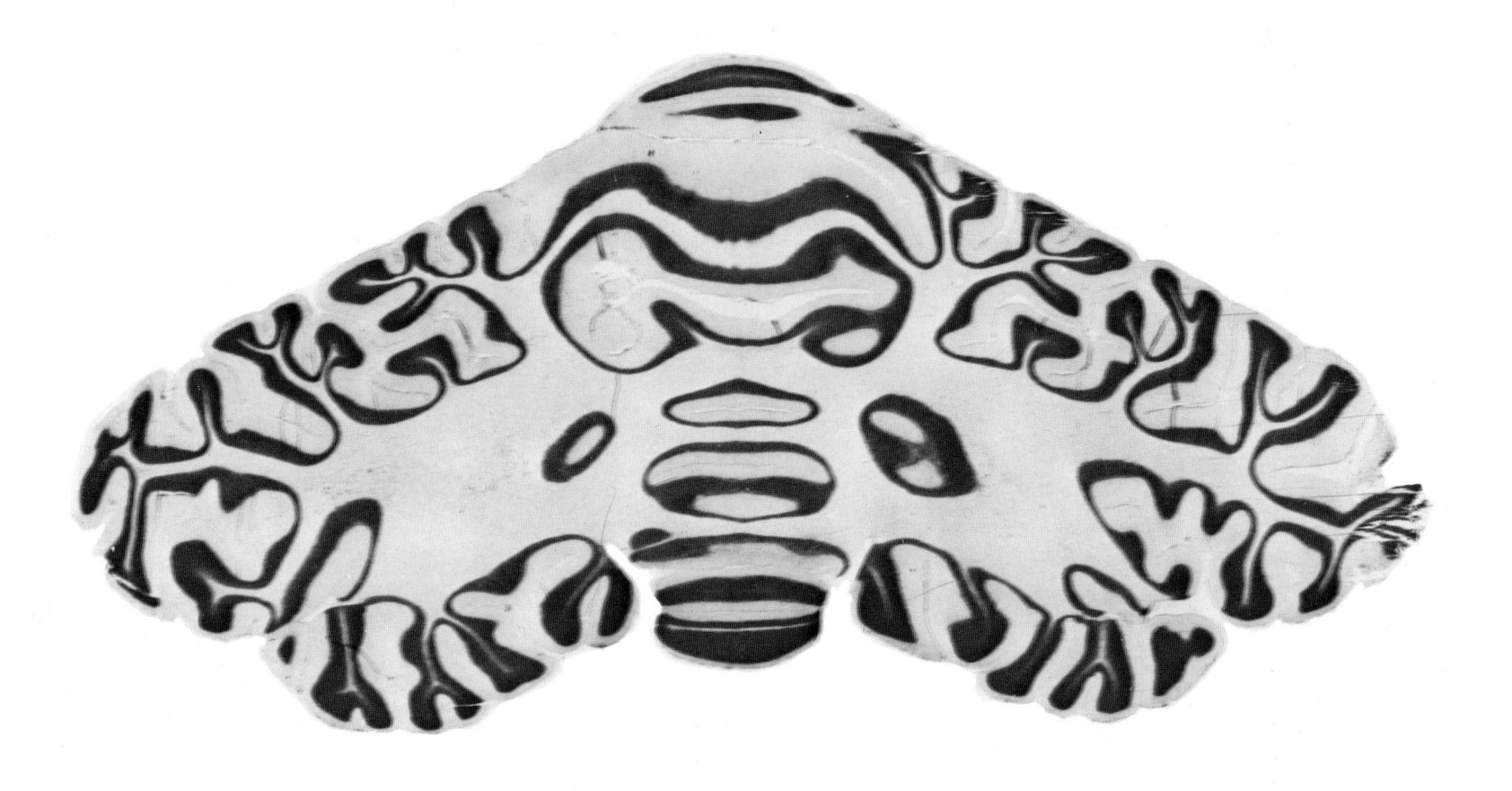

Figs. 101–102 In this section folium VI$_a$ lies within the primary fissure while folium VI$_{b-c}$ occupies the surface. Its continuity from the vermal to the hemispheric portions of the simple lobule is demonstrated.

Both crus I and crus II are prominent in the hemispheres. In the central medullary substance the core of vermal lobule VIII has now separated from the core common to lobules VI and VII, while the uvula (**lobule IX**) is present in the vermis ventrally.

The dorsal paraflocculus is present on the ventral surface of the hemispheres.   *Nissl. X 6*

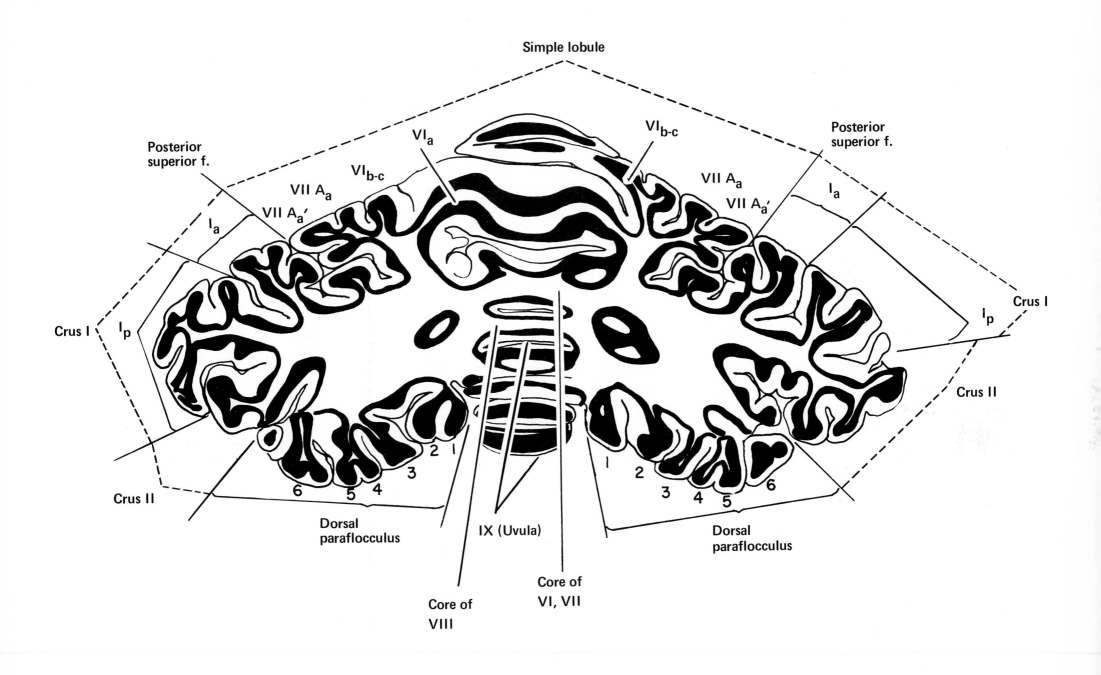

Simple lobule

Posterior superior f.

VI_a

VI_{b-c}

Posterior superior f.

VII A_a

VI_{b-c}

VII A_a

VII A_a'

VII A_a'

I_a

I_a

Crus I

Crus I

I_p

I_p

Crus II

Crus II

2 1

1 2

3

3

6 5 4

4 5 6

Dorsal paraflocculus

Dorsal paraflocculus

Core of VIII

IX (Uvula)

Core of VI, VII

121

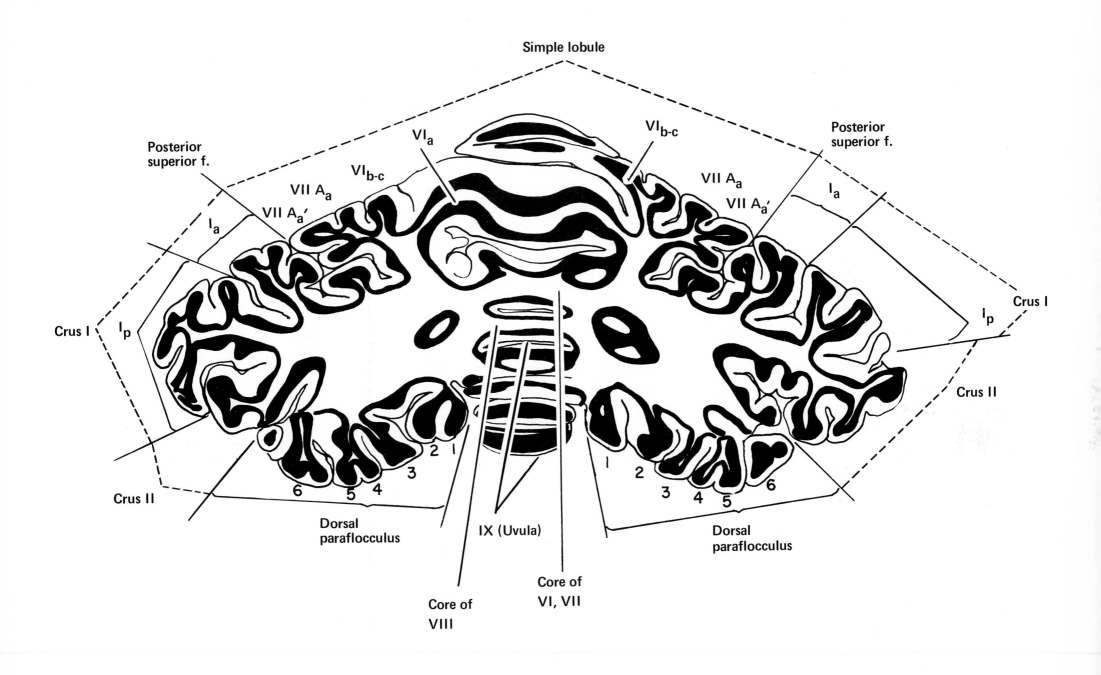

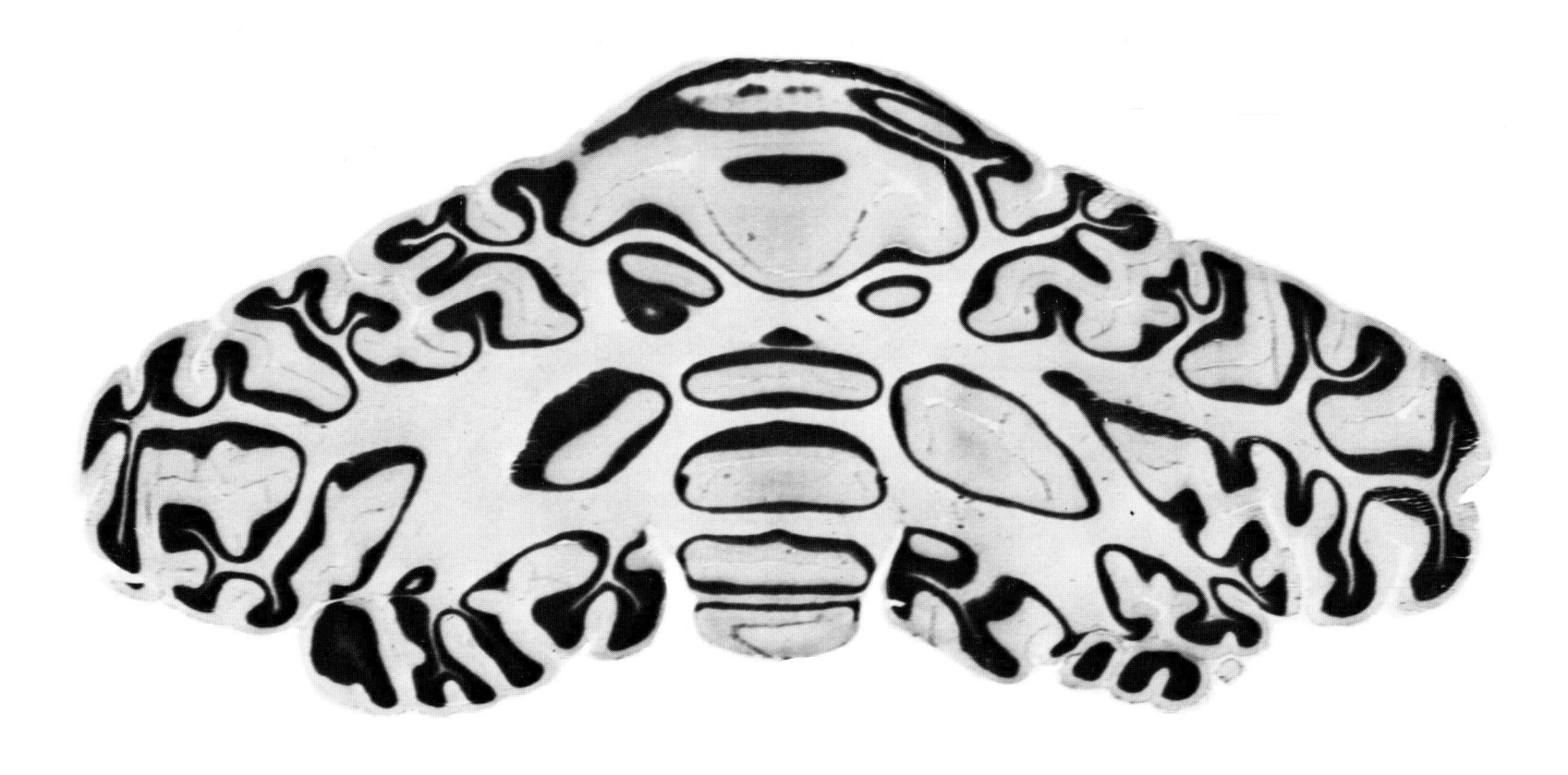

Figs. 103–104 In this section the configuration of the simple lobule is unchanged from that of the previous section. In the hemispheres, crus I_a and I_p are present and crus II is becoming more prominent. On the right, crus II can be seen divided into two subdivisions, crus II_a and II_p. Ventrally, the dorsal paraflocculus has become less prominent in the hemispheres as has the uvula (**lobule IX**) in the vermis.

The core of the vermal lobule VIII and the core of lobules VI and VII, lie unchanged in the central medullary substance.   *Nissl. X 6.*

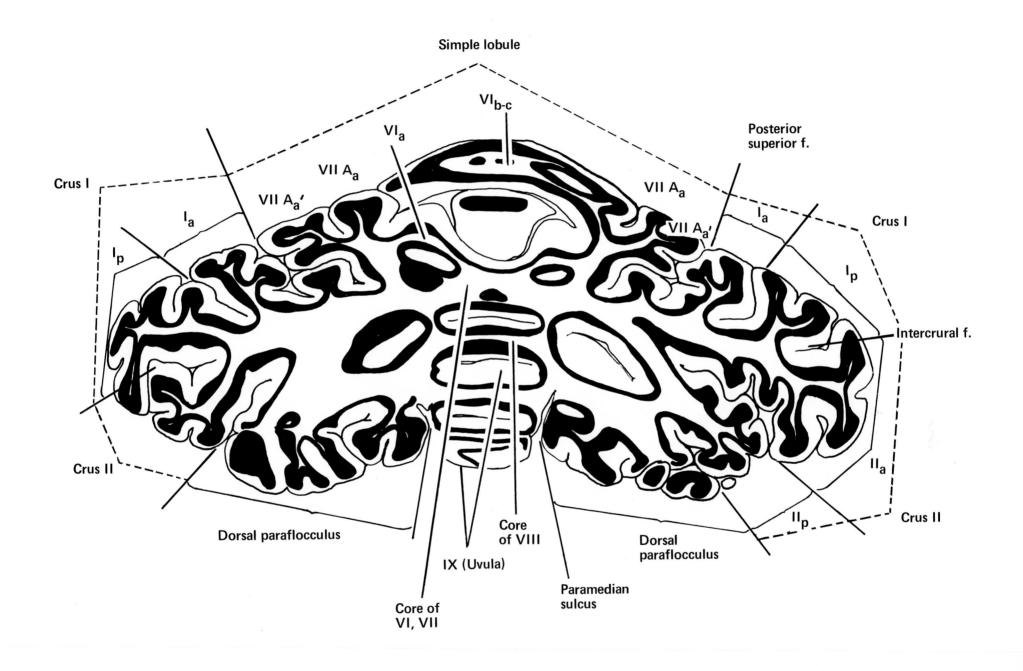

Simple lobule

VI_{b-c}

VI_a

VII A_a

VII A_a'

Posterior superior f.

VII A_a

Crus I

I_a

VII A_a'

I_a

Crus I

I_p

I_p

Intercrural f.

Crus II

II_a

Dorsal paraflocculus

Core of VIII

IX (Uvula)

Dorsal paraflocculus

II_p

Crus II

Paramedian sulcus

Core of VI, VII

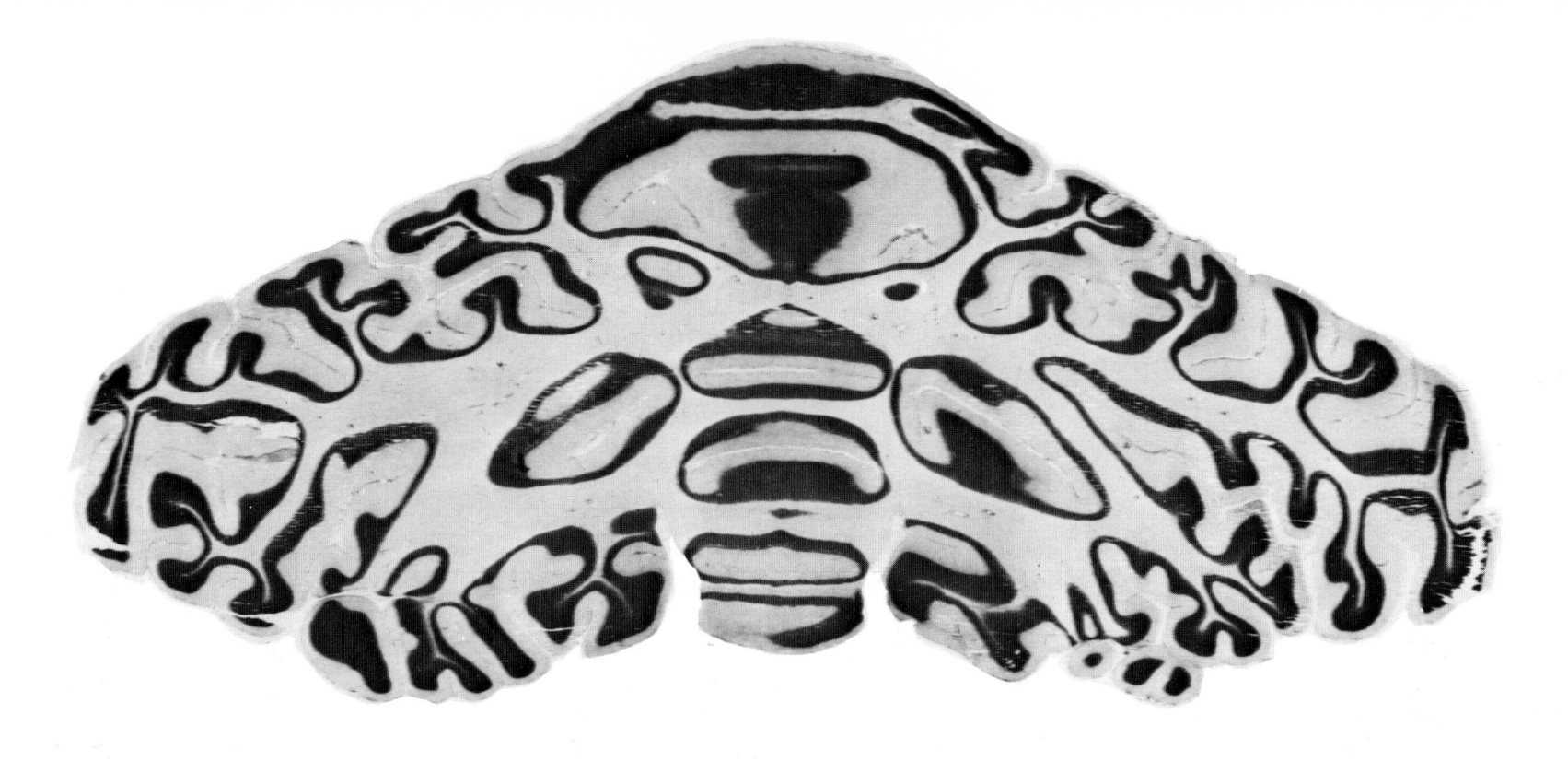

Figs. 105–106   In this section folium VI$_{b-c}$ of the simple lobule extends from the vermis bilaterally into the hemispheres. The remaining portion of the simple lobule in the hemispheres is derived from the single vermal folium VIIA$_a$, and is little changed from the previous section.

The ansiform lobule is now fully developed in the hemispheres, and consists of four divisions: crus I$_a$, crus I$_p$, crus II$_a$, and crus II$_p$.

Ventrally, the uvula (**lobule IX**) is present in the vermis, unchanged from the previous section, while the paramedian lobule is replacing the most caudal folia of the dorsal paraflocculus in the hemispheres.

The core of lobule VIII, the core of lobules VI and VII, and the paramedian sulcus are all unchanged from the previous section.   *Nissl. X 6.*

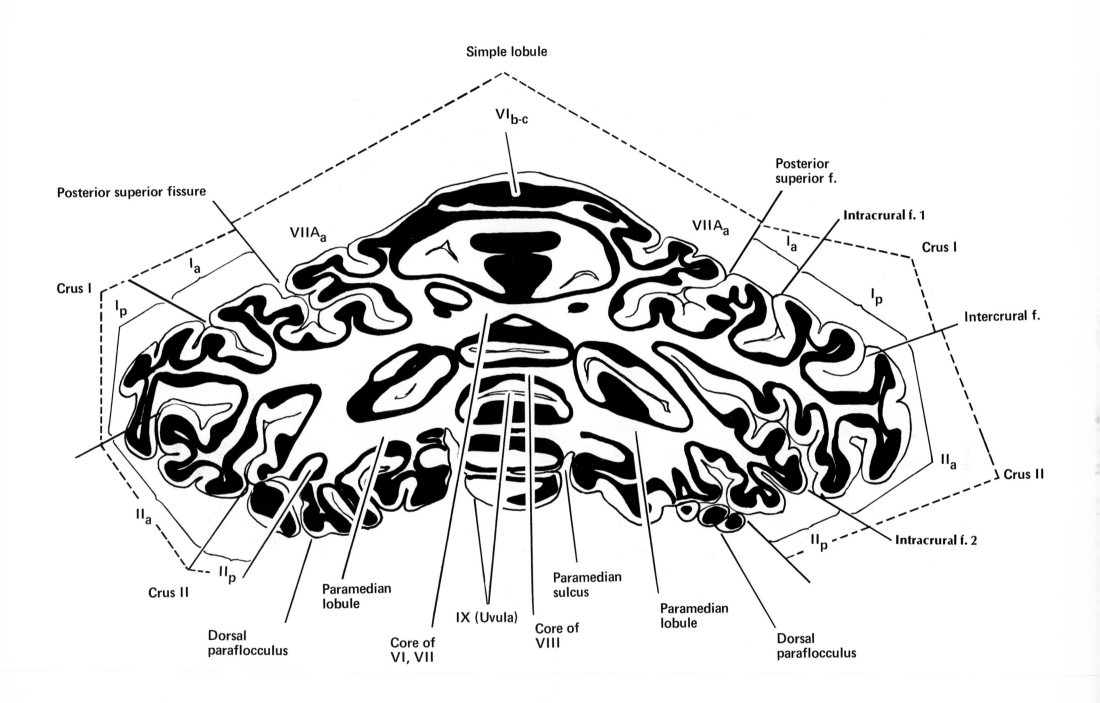

Simple lobule

VI_{b-c}

Posterior superior fissure

Posterior superior f.

$VIIA_a$

$VIIA_a$

Intracrural f. 1

I_a

I_a

Crus I

Crus I

I_p

I_p

Intercrural f.

II_a

Crus II

II_a

II_p

Intracrural f. 2

Crus II

II_p

Paramedian lobule

Paramedian sulcus

Paramedian lobule

Dorsal paraflocculus

Core of VI, VII

IX (Uvula)

Core of VIII

Dorsal paraflocculus

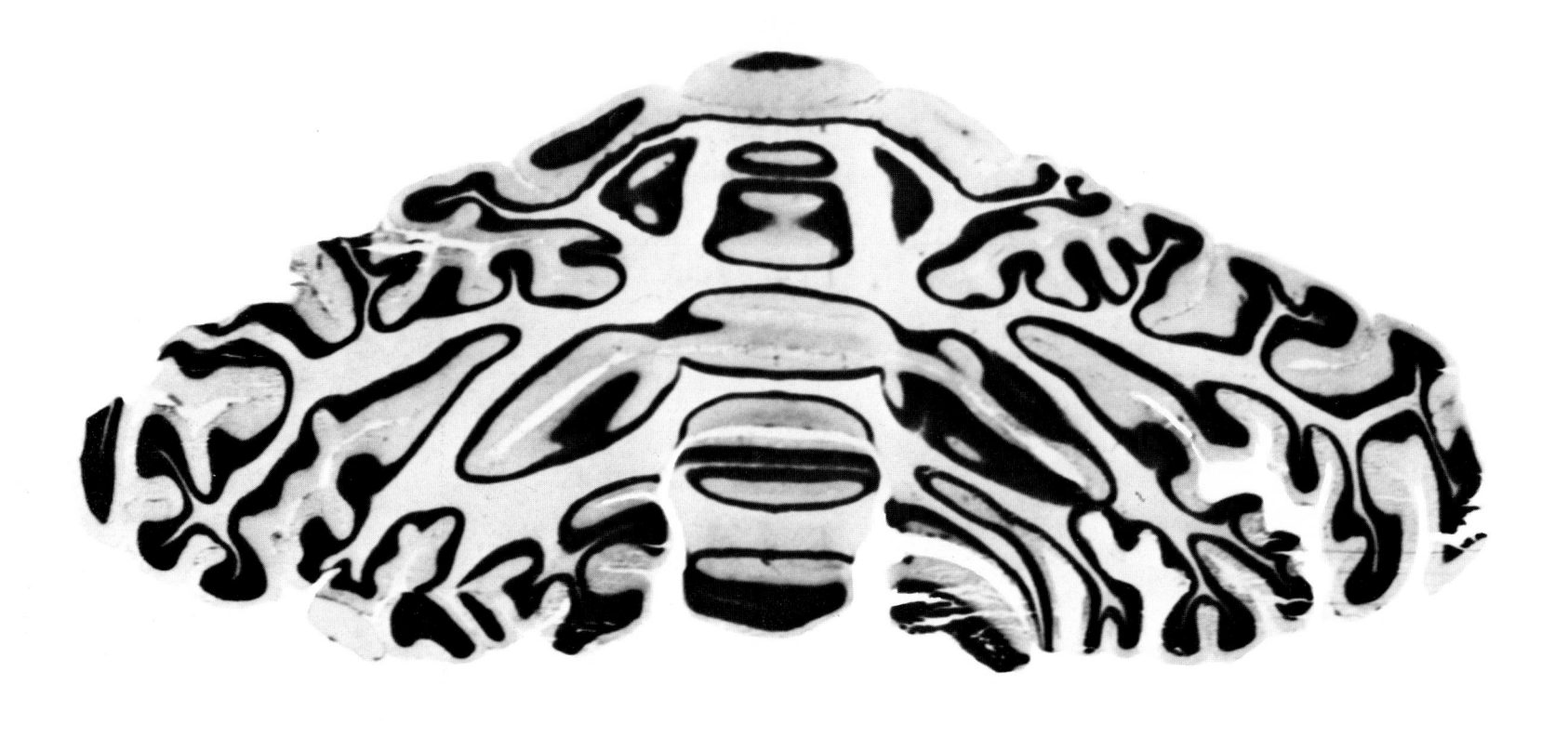

Figs. 107–108 In this section the folia of lobule VI have disappeared and only the most posterior portions of the simple lobule remain. It is clearly demonstrated that folium VIIA$_a$, indicated superiorly in the vermis, extends laterally on both sides to form the posterior folia of the simple lobule in the hemispheres.

As noted in the previous section, the ansiform lobule, with its four divisions, is fully developed in the hemispheres.

The uvula (**lobule IX**) and the core of lobule VIII are unchanged in the vermis, while the paramedian lobule has replaced the dorsal paraflocculus ventrally in the hemispheres.   *Nissl. X 6.*

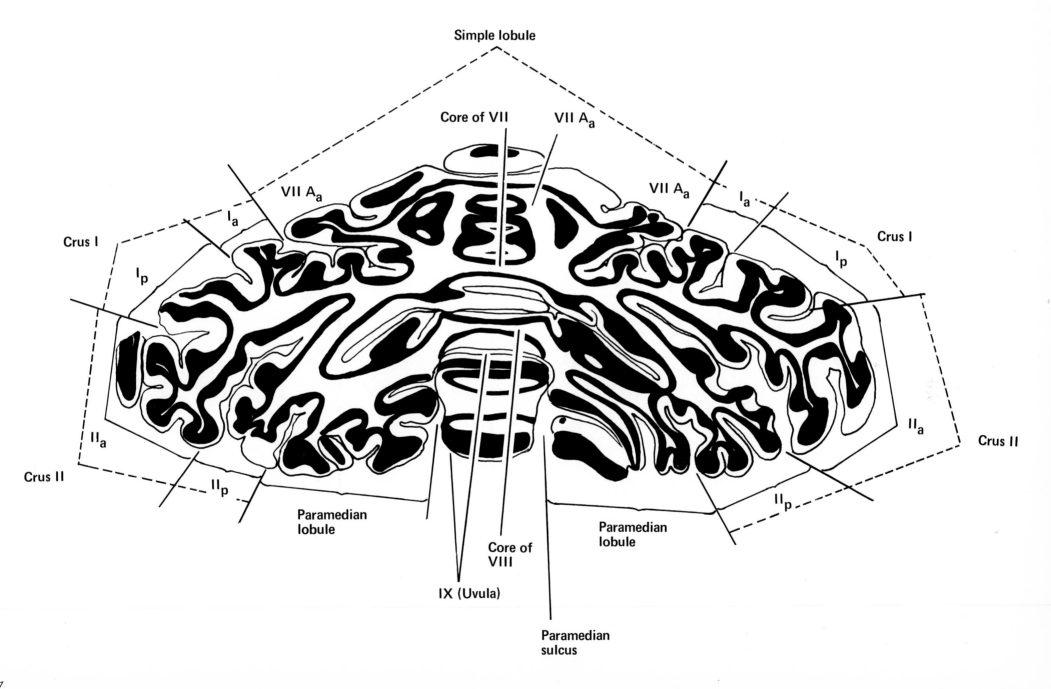

Simple lobule

Core of VII   VII A$_a$

VII A$_a$ VII A$_a$

I$_a$ I$_a$

Crus I   Crus I

I$_p$ I$_p$

II$_a$ II$_a$

Crus II   Crus II

II$_p$ II$_p$

Paramedian lobule   Paramedian lobule

Core of VIII

IX (Uvula)

Paramedian sulcus

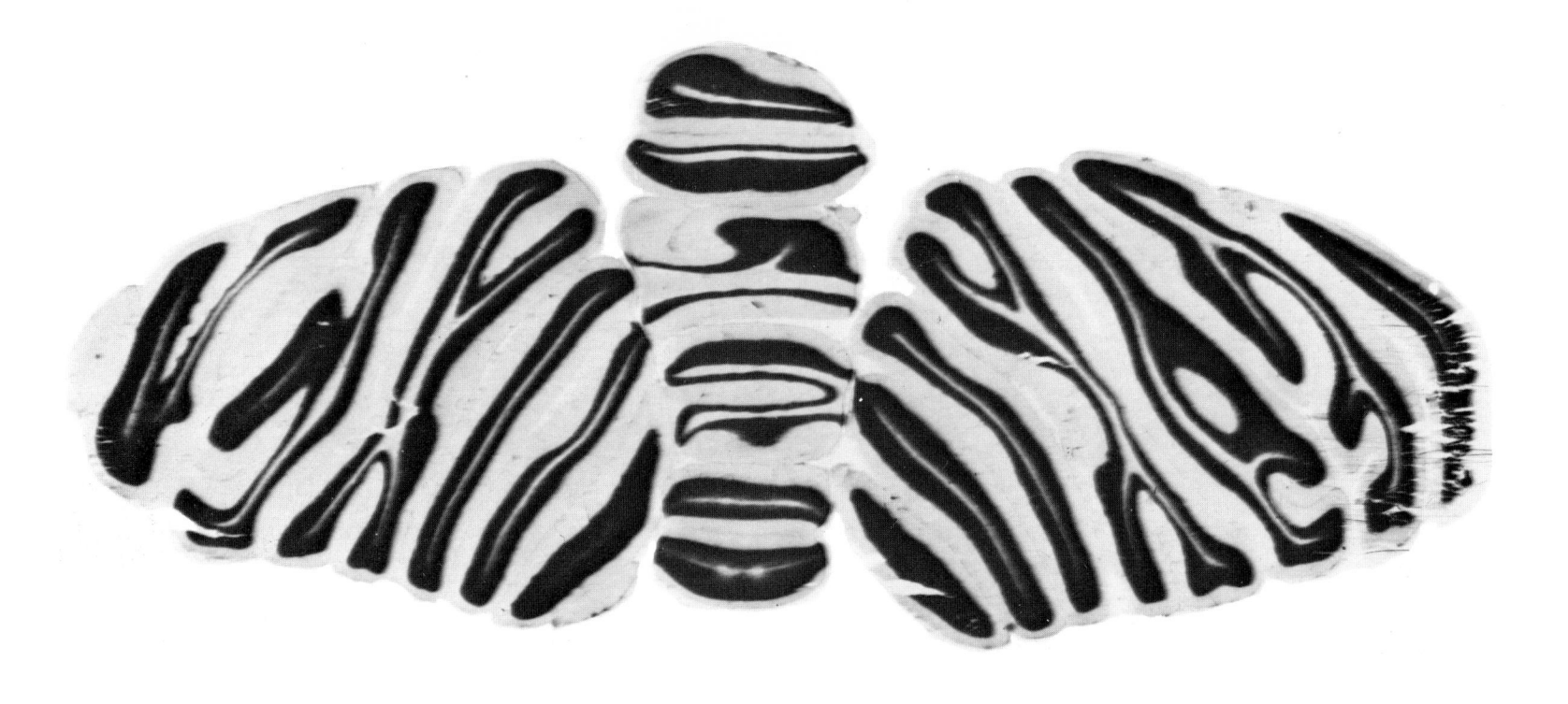

Figs. 109–110 In this section the central medullary core has disappeared and only the more posterior structures of the cerebellum are present.

In the vermis folia VIIA$_b$ and VIIA$_c$ remain dorsally while only two folia of the uvula (**lobule IX**) persist ventrally. Lobule VIII lies in the central vermis and has developed from the medullary core noted in the previous section.

Only crus II$_a$ and crus II$_p$ remain of the ansiform lobule, which occupies the entire lateral extent of the hemispheres.

The medial portion of the hemispheres is now occupied by the paramedian lobule, which has become considerably larger.   *Nissl. X 6.*

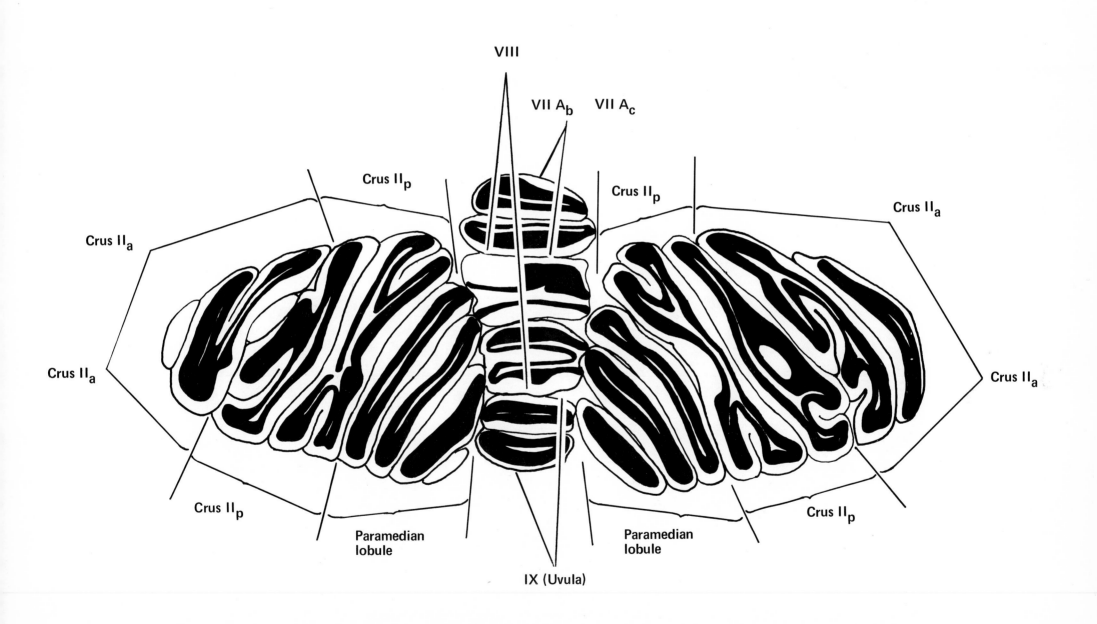

VIII

VII A_b   VII A_c

Crus II_p   Crus II_p

Crus II_a   Crus II_a

Crus II_a   Crus II_a

Crus II_p   Crus II_p

Paramedian   Paramedian
lobule   lobule

IX (Uvula)

129

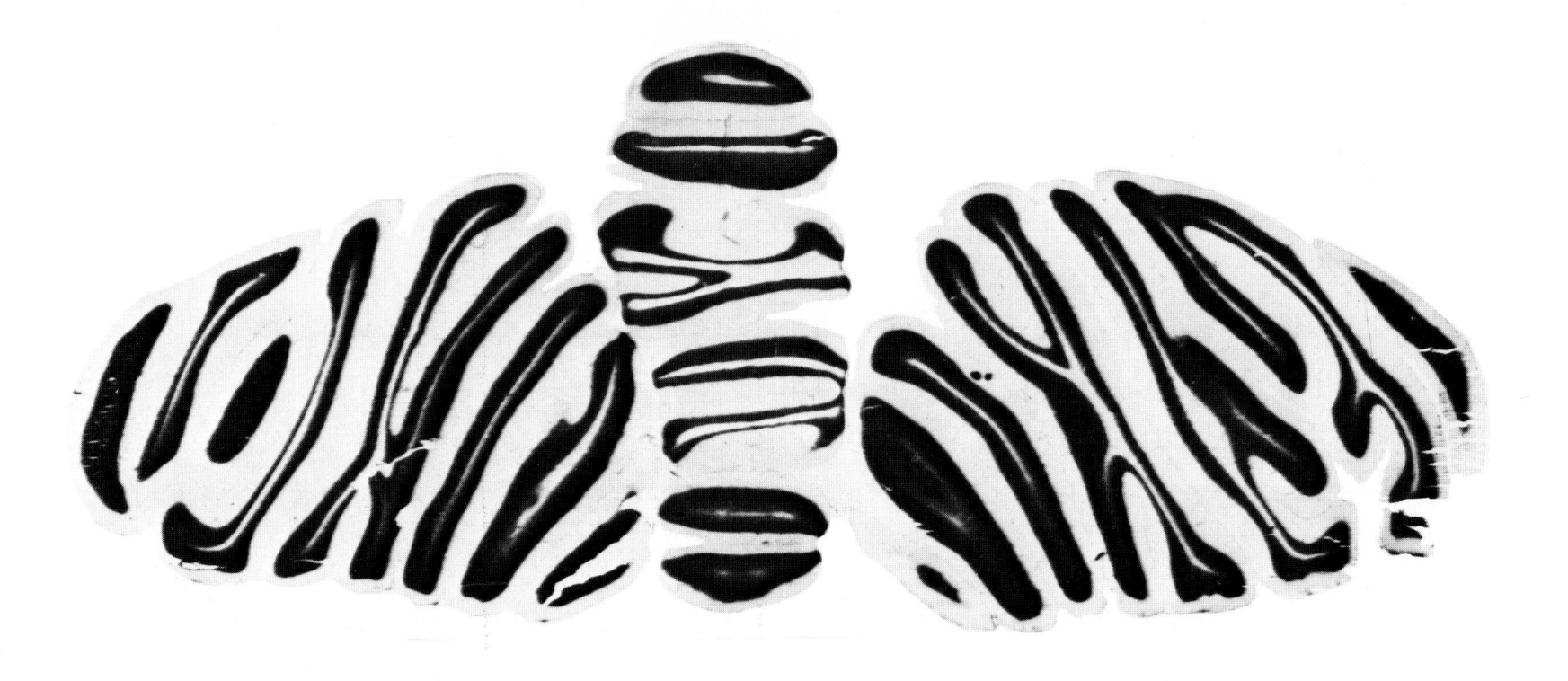

Figs. 111–112   In this section the structures of the vermis, folia VIIA$_b$ and VIIA$_c$, lobule VIII, and the uvula (**lobule IX**), are unchanged.

In the hemispheres the paramedian lobule and crus II$_a$ are reduced in size, while crus II$_p$ is more prominent.   *Nissl. X 6.*

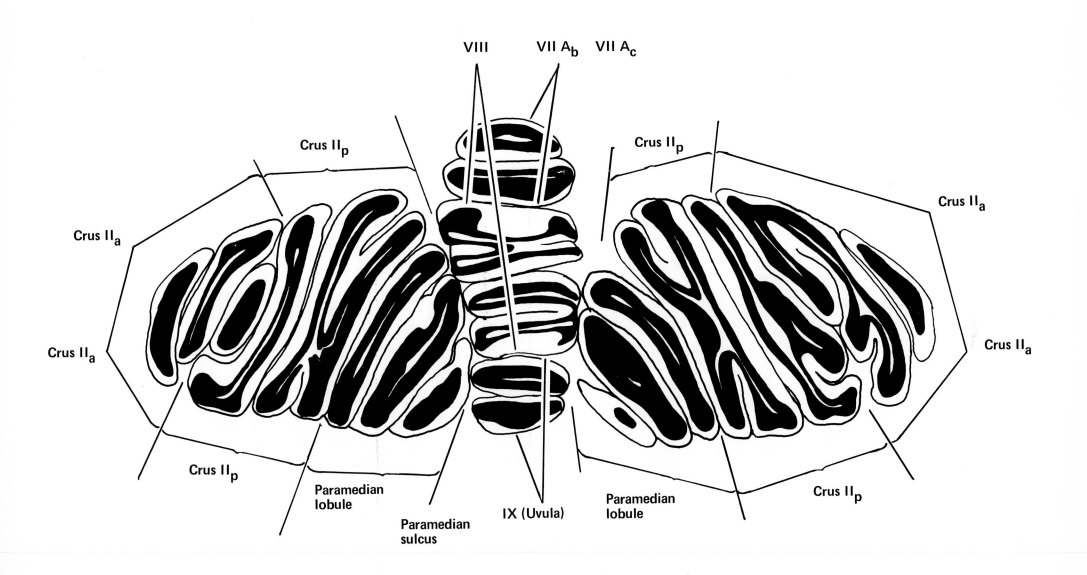

VIII   VII A$_b$ VII A$_c$

Crus II$_p$

Crus II$_p$

Crus II$_a$

Crus II$_a$

Crus II$_a$

Crus II$_a$

Crus II$_p$

Crus II$_p$

Paramedian
lobule

Paramedian
lobule

Paramedian
sulcus

IX (Uvula)

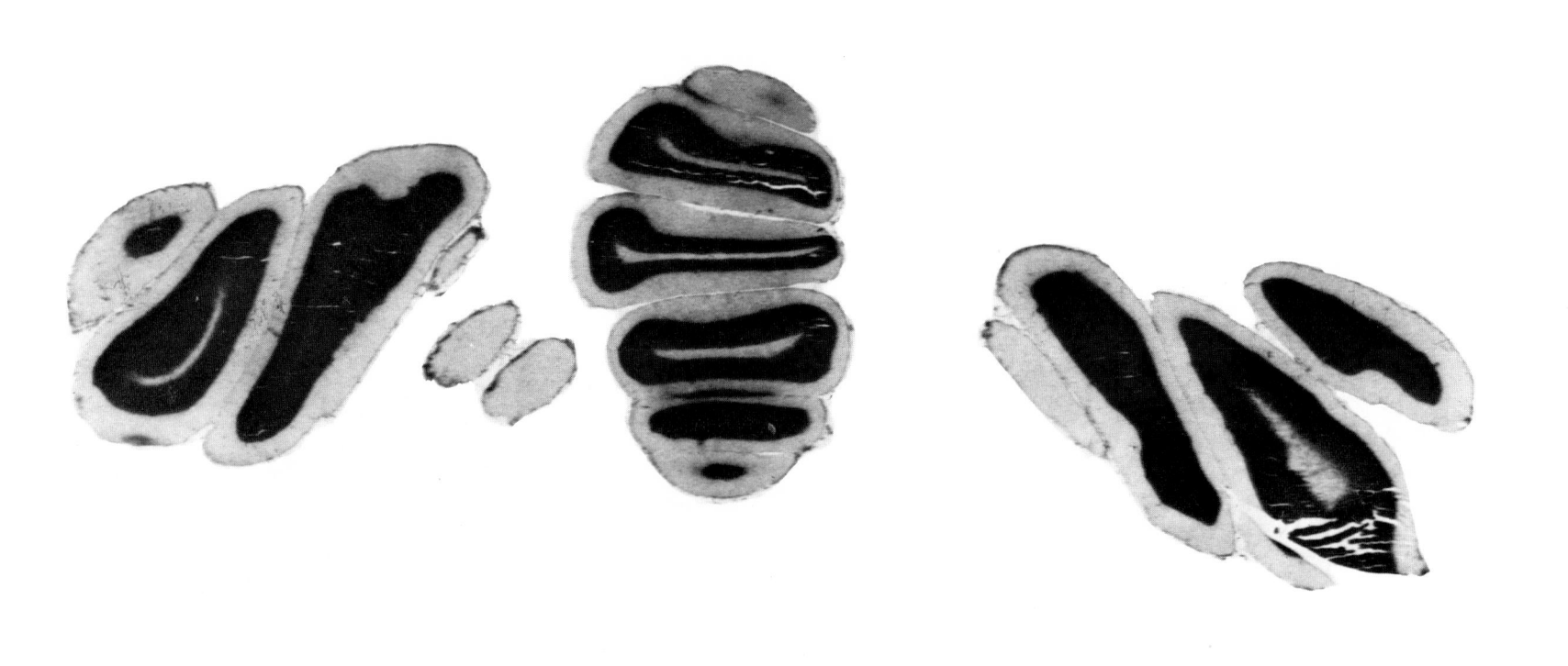

Figs. 115–116   In this most posterior section of the transverse series, only lobule VIII remains in the vermis, while crus II$_p$ is the most prominent structure in the hemispheres.   *Nissl. X 10.*

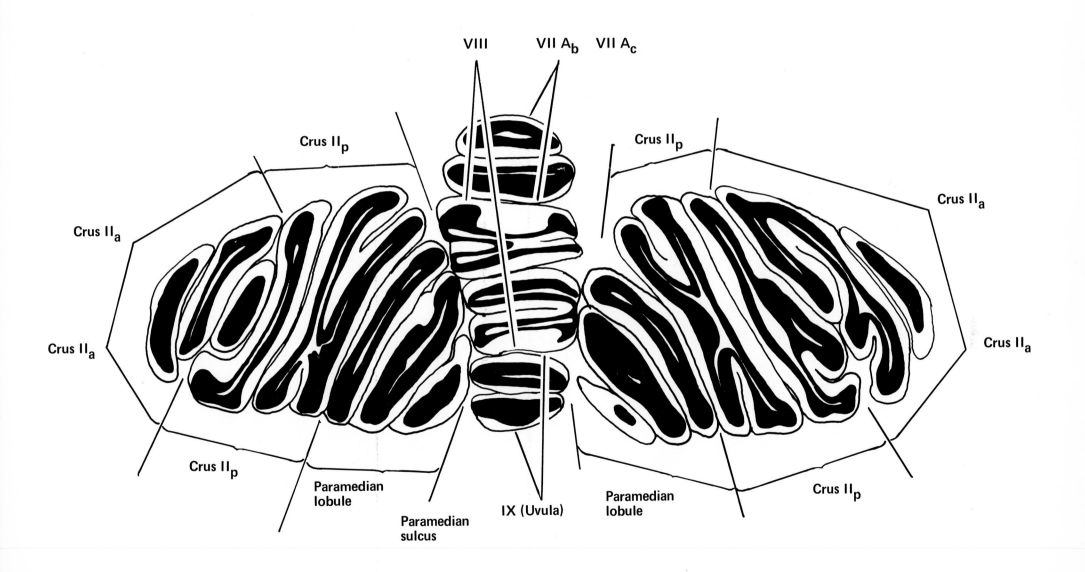

VIII   VII A_b   VII A_c

Crus II_p

Crus II_a

Crus II_a

Crus II_p

Paramedian
lobule

Paramedian
sulcus

IX (Uvula)

Paramedian
lobule

Crus II_p

Crus II_a

Crus II_a

Crus II_p

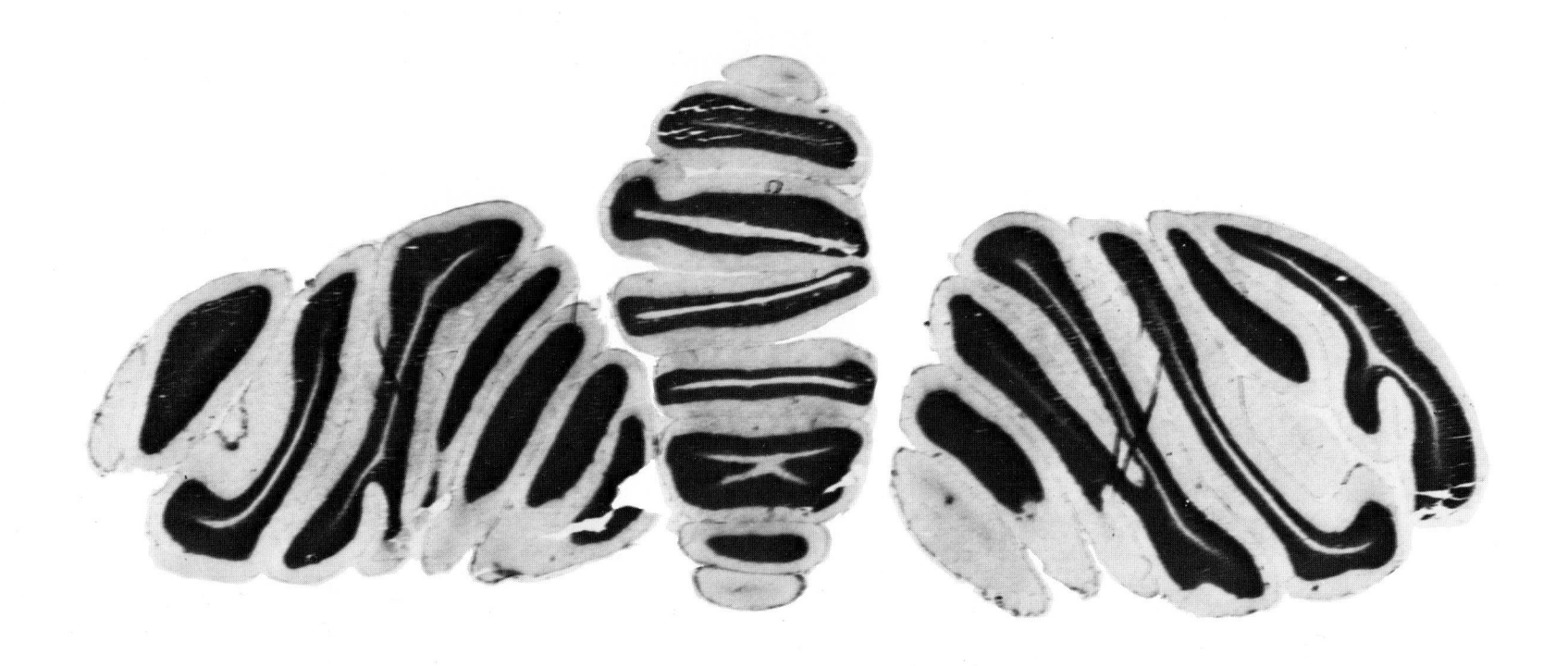

Figs. 113–114 In this section in the vermis folia VIIA$_b$ and VIIA$_c$ and the uvula (**lobule IX**) are greatly reduced in size while lobule VIII is more prominent.

In the hemispheres crus II$_a$ and the paramedian lobule, as in the previous section, are decreasing in size while crus II$_p$ is little changed. *Nissl. X 6.*

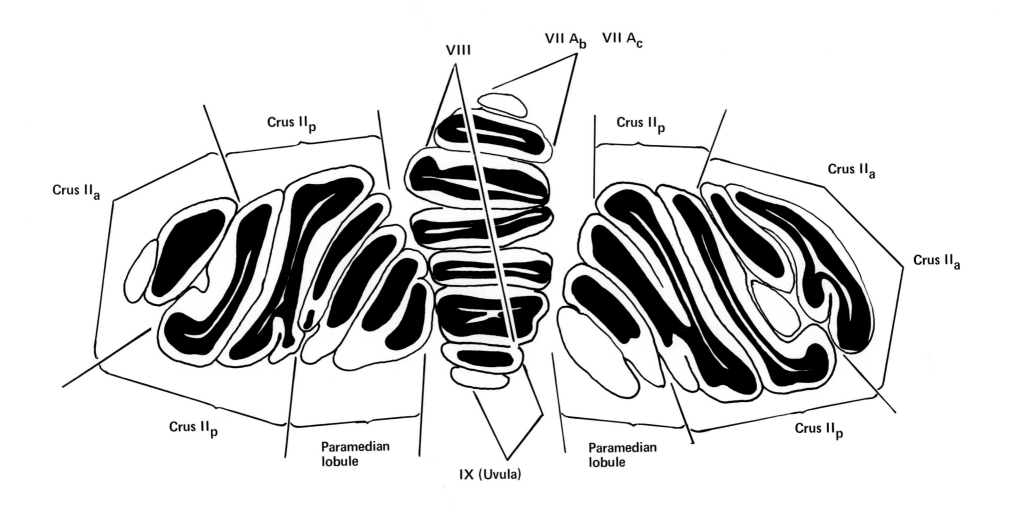

VIII

VII A_b   VII A_c

Crus II_p

Crus II_a

Crus II_p

Crus II_a

Crus II_a

Crus II_p

Paramedian
lobule

Paramedian
lobule

Crus II_p

IX (Uvula)

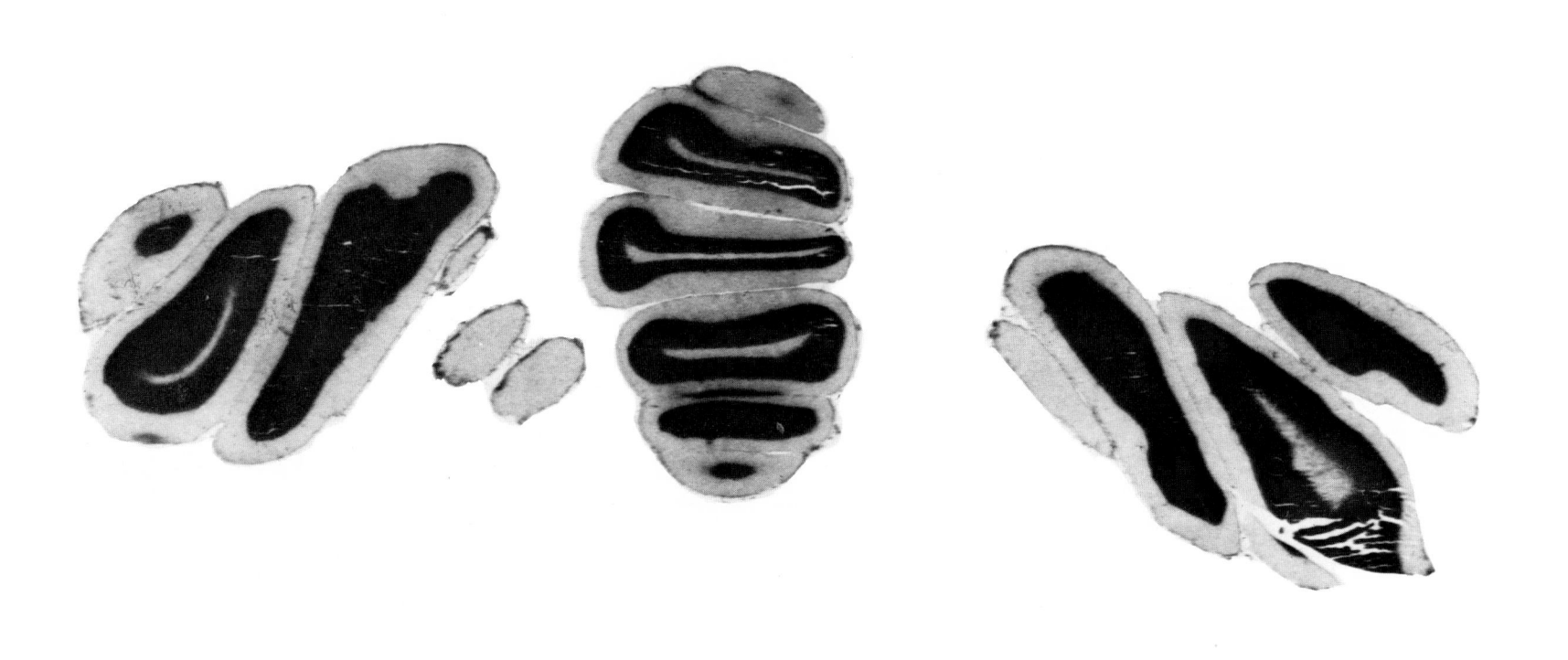

Figs. 115–116 In this most posterior section of the transverse series, only lobule VIII remains in the vermis, while crus II$_p$ is the most prominent structure in the hemispheres.　　*Nissl. X 10.*

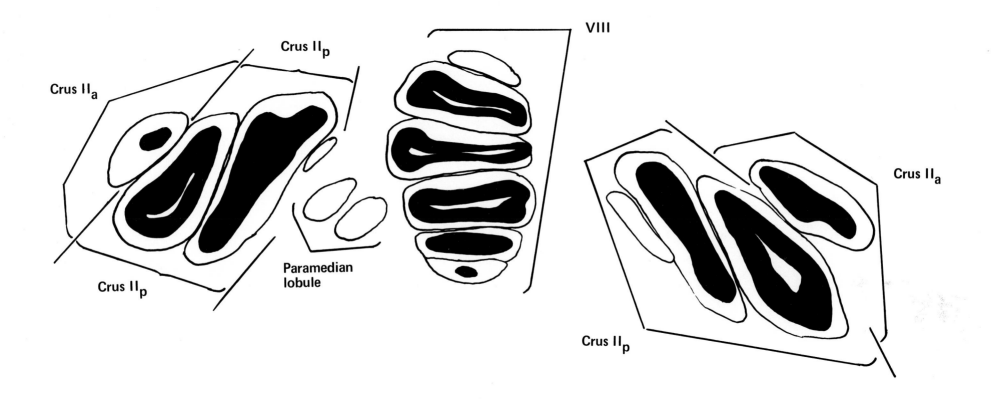

Crus II_a

Crus II_p

Crus II_p

Paramedian
lobule

VIII

Crus II_a

Crus II_p

Bibliography

Bibliography

ANGEVINE, J.B., MANCALL, E.L., and YAKOVLEV, P.I. 1961 The Human Cerebellum. An Atlas of Gross Topography in Serial Sections. Little, Brown and Company, Boston.

BELL, C.C., and DOW, R.S. 1967 Cerebellar circuitry. Neurosci. Res. Progr. Bull., 5: (2) 121–222.

BOLK, L. 1906 Das Cerebellum der Säugethiere. E.F. Bohn, Harlem.

CAJAL, S. RAMÓN y 1909–1911 Histologie du système nerveux de l'homme et des vertébrés. Norbert Maloine, Paris, 2 vols.

COURVILLE, J., and COOPER, C.W. 1970 The cerebellar nuclei of macaca mulatta: A morphological study, J. Comp. Neurol., 140: 241-254.

ECCLES, J.C., ITO, M., and SZENTÁGOTHAI, J. 1967 The Cerebellum as a Neuronal Machine. J. Springer Verlag, New York.

FOX, C.A., HILLMAN, D.E., SIEGESMUND, K.A., and DUTTA, C.R. 1967 The primate cerebellar cortex: A Golgi and electron microscope study. In: C.A. Fox and R.S. Snider (Editors), Progress in Brain Research, The Cerebellum, Vol. 25. Elsevier Publishing Company, Amsterdam, pp. 174–225.

HAMPSON, J.L., HARRISON, C.R., and WOOLSEY, C.N. 1952 Cerebrocerebellar projections and the somatotopic localization of motor function in the cerebellum. Res. Publ. Assn. nerv. ment. Dis., 30: 299–316.

JANSEN, J. 1950 The morphogenesis of the cetacean cerebellum. J. Comp. Neurol., 93: 341–400.

LARSELL, O. 1952 The morphogenesis and adult pattern of the lobules and fissures of the cerebellum of the white rat. J. Comp. Neurol., 97: 281–356.

LARSELL, O. 1953 The cerebellum of the cat and the monkey. J. Comp. Neurol., 99: 135–200.

RILEY, H.A. 1928 The mammalian cerebellum. A comparative study of the arbor vitae and folial pattern. Arch. Neurol. & Psychiat., 20: 895–1034.

SCHEIBEL, M.E., and SCHEIBEL, A.B. 1954 Observations on the intracortical relations of the climbing fibers of the cerebellum. A Golgi study. J. Comp. Neurol., 101: 733–764.

SNIDER, R.S. 1952 Interrelations of cerebellum and brain stem. Res. Publ. Assn. nerv. ment. Dis., 30: 267–281.